KT-198-385

Anaesthesiology: Churchill's Ready Reference

WITHDRAWN FROM LIBRARY

BRITISH MEDICAL ASSOCIATION

0964120

Commissioning Editor: Alison Taylor

Development Editor: Ailsa Laing

Project Manager: Jagannathan Varadarajan

Designer/Design Direction: Stewart Larking

Illustration Manager: Bruce Hogarth

Illustrator: Andrew Bezear

Anaesthesiology
Churchill's **Ready** Reference

Edited by

Michael (Monty) Mythen MBBS FRCA MD
Smiths Medical Professor of Anaesthesia and Critical Care, University College London, London, UK

Edward Burdett MBBS MA MRCP FRCA
Specialist Registrar, Anaesthesia, University College Hospital, London, UK

Robert CM Stephens BA MBBS FRCA
Consultant in Anaesthesia, University College London Hospitals and Research Training Fellow in Anaesthesia, Portex Unit, Institute of Child Health, London, UK

David A Walker BM MRCP FRCA
Consultant in Critical Care Medicine and Anaesthesia, University College London Hospitals, London, UK

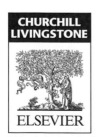

CHURCHILL
LIVINGSTONE

ELSEVIER

Edinburgh London New York Oxford Philadelphia St Louis Sydney Toronto 2010

CHURCHILL
LIVINGSTONE

© 2010, Elsevier Limited. All rights reserved.

No part of this publication may be reproduced or transmitted in any form or by any means, electronic or mechanical, including photocopying, recording, or any information storage and retrieval system, without permission in writing from the publisher. Permissions may be sought directly from Elsevier's Rights Department: phone: (+1) 215 239 3804 (US) or (+44) 1865 843830 (UK); fax: (+44) 1865 853333; e-mail: healthpermissions@elsevier. com. You may also complete your request online via the Elsevier website at http://www. elsevier.com/permissions.

First published 2010

ISBN 978-0-08-045137-4

British Library Cataloguing in Publication Data
A catalogue record for this book is available from the British Library

Library of Congress Cataloging in Publication Data
A catalog record for this book is available from the Library of Congress

Notice

Knowledge and best practice in this field are constantly changing. As new research and experience broaden our knowledge, changes in practice, treatment and drug therapy may become necessary or appropriate. Readers are advised to check the most current information provided (i) on procedures featured or (ii) by the manufacturer of each product to be administered, to verify the recommended dose or formula, the method and duration of administration, and contraindications. It is the responsibility of the practitioner, relying on their own experience and knowledge of the patient, to make diagnoses, to determine dosages and the best treatment for each individual patient, and to take all appropriate safety precautions. To the fullest extent of the law, neither the Publisher nor the Editors assume any liability for any injury and/or damage to persons or property arising out of or related to any use of the material contained in this book.

The Publisher

ELSEVIER your source for books,
journals and multimedia
in the health sciences
www.elsevierhealth.com

Working together to grow
libraries in developing countries
www.elsevier.com | www.bookaid.org | www.sabre.org

ELSEVIER   BOOK AID International   Sabre Foundation

The
Publisher's
policy is to use
paper manufactured
from sustainable forests

Printed in Europe

Contents

Preface   vii
Contributors   ix

Topic 1   **The airway**   1
          Edward Burdett, Anil Patel

Topic 2   **Respiratory system**   8
          Edward Burdett, Robert Stephens, David Walker

Topic 3   **Cardiovascular system**   37
          Kate von Klemperer, David Walker

Topic 4   **Central nervous system**   58
          Caroline Pritchard, Yogi Amin

Topic 5   **Peripheral nervous system**   87
          Caroline Pritchard, Yogi Amin

Topic 6   **Renal, metabolic and endocrine
          systems**   96
          Ramani Moonesinghe

Topic 7   **Haematology and coagulation**   130
          Clare Melikian, Sue Mallett

Topic 8   **The labour ward**   153
          Ruairi Moulding, Roshan Fernando

Topic 9   **Intensive care**   165
          Subodh Tote, Murali Thavasothy

Topic 10 **Therapeutic drug monitoring**   179
          Nicola Hill, Rob Shulman

Preface

The way we manage patients is influenced by the data we receive from investigations; a thorough understanding of the significance of this data is essential. Anaesthetists are unique in that they interact with almost all hospital specialties, and must therefore have a working knowledge of a broad range of investigations.

This book aids the anaesthetist in the correct interpretation of data, and therefore helps in the rational decision-making that is essential to successful outcomes, by giving a brief and practical overview of the many tests that the anaesthetist will come across. The level of detail has been carefully considered, so that only the most pertinent points are given. The book also details the limitations and complications of tests, so that unnecessary investigations and consequent patient anxiety and morbidity may be minimized.

Data from the investigations in this book are not listed exhaustively – rather the entry earns a place if it has relevance to the anaesthetist or the intensive care physician. The book also outlines the physical and physiological principles behind the tests, as well as providing a structure to guide further investigation if necessary.

This book will be useful for all those with an interest in anaesthesia and intensive care medicine; it will help anaesthetists of all levels, especially those preparing for postgraduate examinations.

Professor MG Mythen

Contributors

Yogi Amin BSc MBChB FRCA
Consultant in Neuro Anaesthesia and Neuro Critical Care, The National Hospital of Neurology and Neurosurgery, London and Honorary Senior Lecturer, Institute of Neurology and University College London, UK

Edward Burdett MBBS MA MRCP FRCA
Specialist Registrar, Anaesthesia, University College Hospital, London, UK

Roshan Fernando MBChB FRCA
Consultant Anaesthetist & Honorary Senior Lecturer, Department of Anaesthesia, University College London Hospitals, London, UK

Nicola Hill BPharm MRPharmS Clin Dip MSc Pharm Prac
Divisional Pharmacist, Women and Children's Pharmacy Department, Queen Alexandra Hospital Portsmouth NHS Trust, Portsmouth, UK

Sue Mallett MBBS FRCA
Consultant Anaesthetist, Royal Free Hospital, London, UK

Clare Melikian MBBS MRCP FRCA
Consultant Anaesthesist, Anaesthetic Department, Royal Free Hospital, London, UK

S Ramani Moonesinghe BSc MBBS MRCP FRCA
Consultant, Anaesthetics and Intensive Care, Department of Anaesthetics, University College London Hospitals, London, UK

Ruairi Moulding BSc MBBS FRCA
Visiting Instructor, Department of Anesthesiology, University of Michigan, USA
Specialist Registrar, Anaesthesia, University College Hospital, London, UK

Michael (Monty) Mythen MBBS FRCA MD
Smiths Medical Professor of Anaesthesia and Critical Care, University College London, London Biomedical Research Unit, London, UK

Anil Patel FRCA
Consultant Anaesthetist, Royal National Throat, Nose and Ear Hospital, London, UK

Caroline A Pritchard MA MBBS FRCA
Locum Consultant Anaesthetist, Department of Anaesthesia, University College London Hospitals, London, UK

Rob Shulman BSc Pharm (Hons) Clin Dip Pharm DHCPharm PhD
Lead Pharmacist, Critical Care, Pharmacy Department, University College Hospital, University College London Hospitals NHS Foundation Trust, London, UK

Robert CM Stephens BA MBBS FRCA
Consultant in Anaesthesia, University College London Hospitals and Research Training Fellow in Anaesthesia, Portex Unit, Institute of Child Health, London, UK

Murali Thavasothy BSc MRCP DCH FRCA EDIC
Consultant in Intensive Care Medicine, The Royal London Hospital, London, UK

Subodh P Tote MBBS MRCP FRCA EDIC
Consultant Intensive Care Medicine and Anaesthetics, Frimley Park Hospital, Frimley, Surrey, UK

Kate L von Klemperer MBBsh MRCP
Cardiology Registrar, University College London Hospital, London, UK

David A Walker BM MRCP FRCA
Consultant in Critical Care Medicine and Anaesthesia, University College London Hospitals, London, UK

TOPIC ❶

The airway

Topic Contents

Predicting difficult airway management 1
Test: Bedside tests **1**
View at laryngoscopy 4
Test: Cormack and Lehane view **4**

Other investigations of the airway 5
Test: Soft tissue imaging of the lower airway **5**
Test: Flexible nasendoscopy **5**
Test: Flow volume loops **5**
Test: Plain radiography **6**

Predicting difficult airway management

Test: Bedside tests

Indications

Used to predict difficult facemask ventilation and tracheal intubation. They should form part of the routine clinical examination of the patient during the anaesthetist's preoperative assessment, and should be performed in conjunction with a full history and physical examination as appropriate. The latter will not be discussed further in this topic.

Failed intubation and ventilation leading to serious morbidity or death is generally accepted as having an incidence of 1 in 10 000 to 1 in 100 000 of the general surgical population.

The most commonly used tests are listed below.

Mallampati test

First described in 1984 as a three-point scoring system. A modification by Samsoon and Young into a four-point system has generally been accepted.

How it is done

Keeping the head in a neutral position the patient is asked to open the mouth fully and protrude the tongue as far as possible, without phonation. Looking from the patient's eye level the pharyngeal structures are inspected (Fig. 1.1). It has been suggested that the specificity and positive predictive value of the modified Mallampati test is improved by slightly extending the neck.

Interpretation

The following structures are visible:
Class I – soft palate, fauces, uvula, anterior and posterior pillars
Class 2 – soft palate, fauces and uvula
Class 3 – soft palate and the base of the uvula
Class 4 – soft palate is not visible at all.

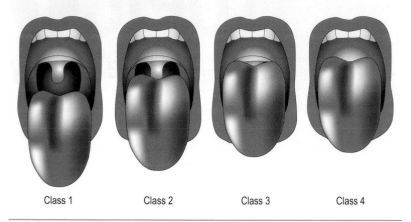

| Class 1 | Class 2 | Class 3 | Class 4 |

Fig. 1.1 Modified Mallampati classification.

Management principles
A prediction of a difficult airway may trigger an alternative management strategy, for example inhalational induction, fibre-optic intubation or awake percutaneous approach under local anaesthesia.

Limitations and complications
- There is no universally accepted definition of what constitutes difficult airway management, which is itself subject to the expertise of the anaesthetist. It can be defined according to time taken, attempts made, hypoxaemia or requirement for a second dose of muscle relaxant.
- Because true failed airway management is very rare (1 in 3000 of the general surgical population), none of the commonly used bedside tests are reliably able to identify those at risk of difficult airway management without a high false negative rate.
- Used alone, therefore, the Mallampati test has limited accuracy for predicting the difficult airway and its use as a screening tool has been called into question. It is undoubtedly valuable when used in conjunction with other bedside tests.

Protrusion of the mandible
This gives an indication of the mobility of the mandible. This can be graded as follows:
Grade A – able to protrude lower teeth beyond upper incisors
Grade B – able to protrude lower teeth until they are level with upper teeth
Grade C – not able to oppose upper and lower incisors.

If the patient is grade A or B, intubation is usually straightforward. If the patient cannot get the upper and lower incisors into alignment intubation is more likely to be difficult.

Thyromental and sternomental distance
To obtain thyromental distance the patient is asked to fully extend the neck from neutral position. The distance from the mentum to the thyroid notch is measured. A distance of less than 6 cm is associated with difficult laryngoscopy.

Sternomental distance is measured from the sternum to the tip of the mandible with the head extended and is influenced by a number of factors including neck extension. It has also been noted to be a useful screening test for preoperative prediction of difficult intubation. A sternomental distance of 12.5 cm or less predicts difficult intubation.

Head extension

Keeping the head in a neutral position and the line joining the mentum to the angle of the mandible parallel to the floor, the patient is asked to maximally extend the head on the neck. The angle traversed by the mento-mandibular line is measured. Head extension of 35 degrees or more is normal (Fig. 1.2).

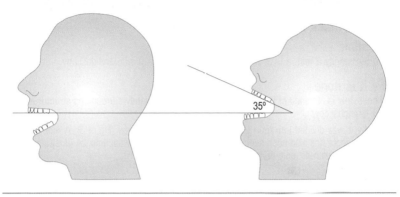

Fig. 1.2 Head extension.

Specifically, extension at the atlanto-axial joint should be assessed by asking the patient to flex their neck by putting their head forward and down. The neck is then held in this position and the patient attempts to raise their face up testing for extension of the atlanto-axial joint. Since laryngoscopy is optimally performed with the neck flexed and extension at the atlanto-axial joint, reduction of movement at this joint is associated with difficulty.

Palm print test

This test is said to predict difficult direct laryngoscopy in diabetic patients, perhaps because it is a marker of small joint stiffness. The palm and fingers of the dominant hand of the patient are painted with ink. The patient then presses the hand firmly against a white sheet of paper on a hard surface. The less that the phalanges are able to touch the paper, the more difficult intubation is likely to be.

Mouth opening

Less than 4 cm is associated with difficult direct laryngoscopy.

Further investigations

These tests can be used in conjunction with other clinical data such as age, gender and body mass index (BMI) to further refine the prediction of difficult ventilation, intubation and laryngoscopy. A variety of these multivariate tests exist, all more sensitive and specific than a simple Mallampati score, but none have been proven to have overall superiority.

LEMON: Stands for look-evaluate-Mallampati-obstruction-neck. It has been used in the USA in a resuscitation setting.

Wilson's risk index: Parameters include weight, head and neck movement, jaw opening and protrusion, buck teeth and receding mandible.

El-Ganzouri risk index: Evaluates mouth opening, thyromental distance, Mallampati, neck movement, jaw protrusion, body weight and history of difficult intubation.

Arne risk index: Devised and validated with patients undergoing ear nose and throat (ENT) surgery, the index scores according to Mallampati score, mouth opening, jaw protrusion, head and neck movement, history of difficult intubation and clinical symptoms.

View at laryngoscopy

Test: Cormack and Lehane view

Indication

While not strictly a test, it is used as a marker of view at direct laryngoscopy.

How it is done

The best view is obtained of the laryngeal inlet and immediately surrounding structures using direct laryngoscopy.

Originally it was divided into four grades, depending on the view (Fig. 1.3). A modified five-grade score has also been suggested, where grade 2 is divided into 2A (posterior border of cords seen) and 2B (only arytenoids and epiglottis seen).

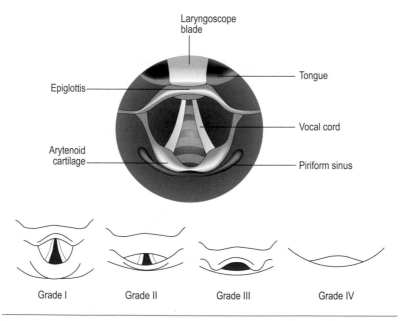

Fig. 1.3 Cormack and Lehane classification of the view at laryngoscopy; anatomy of the glottic opening seen from the pharynx.

Interpretation

Laryngeal view:

Grade I – vocal cords visible

Grade II – only posterior commissure or arytenoids visible

Grade III – only epiglottis visible

Grade IV – no glottic structure visible.

Grade III and IV laryngoscopic views are considered as difficult laryngoscopy as no part of the glottis is visible.

Limitations and complications

- View at laryngoscopy depends on the skill of the operator, and the range of alternative direct laryngoscopy equipment available.
- A poor (grade 3 or 4) view does not always predict difficult intubation, which is after all usually the goal during laryngoscopy.
- The scoring system does not give any guidance as to which alternative technique to facilitate endotracheal intubation would be most appropriate.

Other investigations of the airway

Test: Soft tissue imaging of the lower airway

Indication

Usually in the elective setting when a lower airway abnormality is suspected, either a mass protruding into the airway, or previous surgery or radiotherapy.

How it is done

Computed tomography (CT) or magnetic resonance imaging (MRI) imaging is performed of the upper thorax and neck. This is particularly useful if a mediastinal mass has been diagnosed on plain chest radiography, and the degree of tracheal involvement or invasion must be found.

Limitations and complications

- These investigations are not performed in the acutely unwell patient.
- Rapidly growing pathologies of the mediastinum can quickly render the investigations out-of-date.

Test: Flexible nasendoscopy

Indication

Before elective surgery when anatomical abnormality of structures above the vocal cords is suspected. This is sometimes performed before ENT surgery.

How it is done

It is usually carried out by ENT surgeons. After topical local anaesthesia, a small (<4 mm) endoscope is passed nasally and directed towards the vocal cords. Photographs are taken of abnormal structures, which can be used to plan anaesthesia and oxygenation for elective surgery.

Test: Flow volume loops

See Topic 2.

Test: Plain radiography

Various studies have been used to try to predict difficult intubation by assessing the anatomy of the mandible on x-ray. These have shown that the depth of the mandible may be important, but they are not commonly used as a screening test.

Patients with known conditions affecting the cervical spine, such as rheumatoid arthritis or ankylosing spondylitis should undergo lateral cervical spine radiography before intubation if at all possible. Flexion and extension views are particularly useful in this scenario (Fig. 1.4), both to detect poor neck mobility and consequent difficult direct laryngoscopy, and to pick up potentially unstable ligamentous pathology at the atlanto-axial joint.

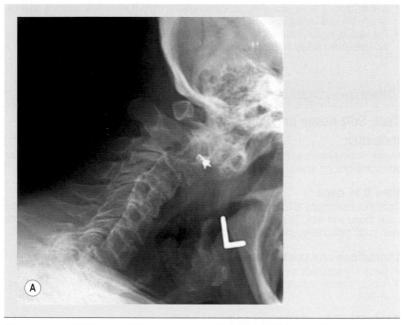

Fig. 1.4 Cervical (A) flexion and (B) extension views of a patient with rheumatoid arthritis. Note the metal pin at the atlanto-axial junction.

(Continued)

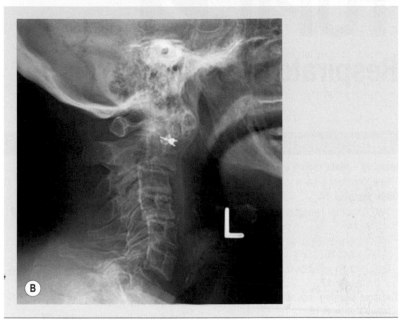

Fig. 1.4 cont'd.

TOPIC ❷

Respiratory system

Topic Contents

Imaging – Plain radiography 8
Test: The chest x-ray 8
Other imaging 14
Test: Computed tomography (CT) scan 14
Test: Ventilation-perfusion scan (VQ scan) 16
Test: Positron emission tomography (PET) scan 17
Thoracic imaging modality in the trauma patient 18
Pulmonary function tests 18
Test: Functional residual capacity 18

Test: Volume/time curve 19
Test: Flow/volume curve (dynamic) 21
Test: Transfer factor/diffusing capacity 25
Intraoperative respiratory monitoring 26
Test: Pulse oximetry (SpO₂) 26
Test: Capnography 26
Test: Shunt fraction 30
Pressure-volume (P/V) curve analysis 31
Test: Static airway compliance 31
Blood gas analysis 33
Test: Arterial blood gas analysis 33

Imaging – Plain radiography

Test: The chest x-ray

Indications

A 'routine' preoperative chest x-ray (CXR) is not necessary unless there are specific indications (see NICE Guidelines1). Management is changed as a result of less than 1% of preoperative films, increasing as the American Society of Anaesthesiologists (ASA) score rises. Acute change in cardiac/respiratory signs or symptoms is the only undisputed indication in elective nonthoracic surgery. Similarly there seems to be no clear advantage to a 'routine' chest x-ray in the intensive care unit (ICU).

The chest x-ray is an essential part of the trauma series and is considered an important adjunct in the diagnosis of chest wall fractures, pneumothorax, haemothorax, and injuries to the heart and great vessels.

How it is done

The standard view is the posteroanterior (PA) film, with the patient facing the cassette and the x-ray tube 2 m away. An anteroposterior (AP) film is taken when the patient is unable to stand, with the cassette behind the patient. In the AP chest x-ray the heart will be magnified, and it is inappropriate to comment on cardiomegaly (unless it is gross) on this basis. A PA view shows the scapulae clear of the lungs whilst in AP they always overlap.

Interpretation

The chest x-ray (Fig. 2.1) is a two-dimensional representation of a three-dimensional structure. An understanding of chest anatomy is essential to interpretation of plain chest x-ray abnormalities.

Owing to the routine use of CT scanning, the lateral chest x-ray and decubitus film are now rarely seen. A lateral x-ray may differentiate structures that are unclear on PA chest x-ray. A decubitus film is taken with the patient on his or her side to assess:

(1) The volume and mobility of a pleural effusion on the dependent side
(2) A suspected pneumothorax in the nondependent side in a patient who cannot be examined erect.

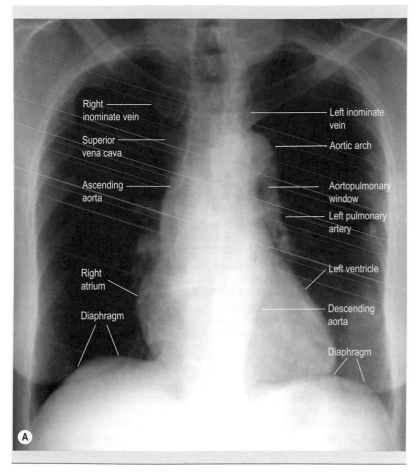

Fig. 2.1 Posteroanterior chest x-ray (A) with diagrammatic annotation (B). The hilum is higher on the left but the hemidiaphragm is lower. The carina is at T4 on expiration and T6 on inspiration.

(Continued)

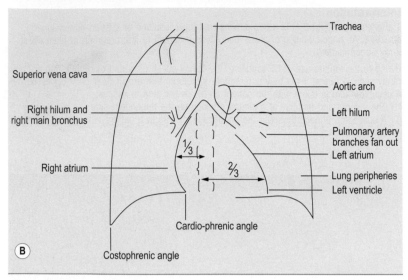

Fig. 2.1 cont'd.

Abnormalities of the lung

Consolidation – infiltration of the alveolar space by inflammatory tissue. The classic example is pneumonia – airspace disease and consolidation, which is not usually associated with volume loss. There may be an associated (parapneumonic) effusion.

The silhouette sign – an interface between isodense structures in contact with each other. The radiographic distinction between anatomical borders of lung and soft tissue can be 'lost' by abnormalities of the lung, which increase its density.

Air bronchogram – when the air spaces fill with pus or fluid, the alveoli fill first with the bronchi being relatively spared, therefore the bronchi stand out. This is called an air bronchogram and is a sign of airspace disease such as consolidation, pulmonary oedema or atelectasis.

Atelectasis: a linear increased density and volume loss on chest x-ray. Some indirect signs of volume loss include vascular crowding or mediastinal shift towards the collapse. There may be compensatory hyperinflation of adjacent lobes, or hilar elevation (upper lobe collapse) or depression (lower lobe collapse).

Interstitial disease

The interstitial space surrounds bronchi, vessels and groups of alveoli. Disease in the interstitium manifests itself by *reticulonodular* shadowing (criss cross lines or tiny nodules or both). The main two processes affecting the interstitium are accumulation of fluid (pulmonary oedema) and inflammation leading to fibrosis (Fig. 2.2 and Box 2.1).

Pulmonary oedema may be cardiogenic or noncardiogenic. In congestive heart failure, the pulmonary capillary wedge pressure (PCWP) rises and the upper zone veins dilate – this is called upper zone blood diversion. With increasing PCWP, interstitial oedema occurs with the appearance of Kerley B lines and prominence of the interlobar fissures. Increased PCWP above this level causes alveolar oedema, often in a classic perihilar 'bat wing' pattern. Pleural effusions also occur. Unusual patterns may be found in patients with chronic obstructive pulmonary disease (COPD) who have predominant upper lobe emphysema.

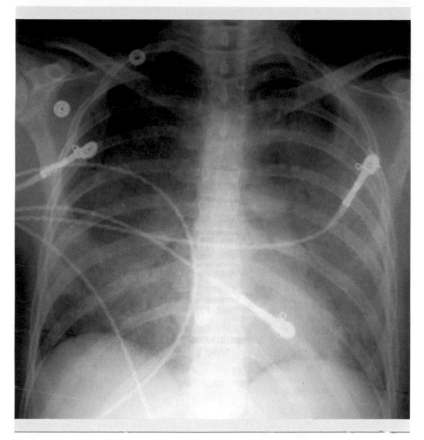

Fig. 2.2 Pulmonary oedema: diffuse hazy shadowing in a bat-wing distribution and upper lobe blood diversion.

Box 2.1 The most common causes of interstitial fibrosis are:

- Idiopathic (IPF, >50% of cases)
- Collagen vascular disease
- Cytotoxic agents and nitrofurantoin
- Pneumoconioses
- Radiation
- Sarcoidosis

A helpful mnemonic for noncardiogenic pulmonary oedema is NOT CARDIAC: **n**ear-drowning, **o**xygen therapy, **t**ransfusion or **t**rauma, **C**NS disorder, **A**RDS, **a**spiration, or **a**ltitude **s**ickness, **r**enal disorder, **d**rugs, **i**nhaled toxins, **a**llergic alveolitis, **c**ontrast or **c**ontusion.

COPD is often seen on CXR as diffuse hyperinflation with flattening of diaphragms and enlargement of pulmonary arteries and right ventricle (cor pulmonale). In smokers the upper lung zones are commonly diseased.

Abnormalities of the mediastinum

On the PA film, the heart takes up to half of the total thoracic measurement in adults (more in children).

In mediastinal deviation, tension pneumothorax and pleural effusion push the mediastinum away; lung collapse pulls it towards the affected side.

Findings for *pneumomediastinum* include streaky lucencies over the mediastinum that extend into the neck and elevation of the parietal pleura along the mediastinal borders.

Causes of pneumomediastinum include:
- Asthma
- Surgery (postoperative complication)
- Traumatic tracheobronchial rupture
- Abrupt changes in intrathoracic pressure (vomiting, coughing, exercise, parturition)
- Ruptured oesophagus
- Barotrauma
- Crack cocaine.

Pericardial effusion causes a globular enlarged heart shadow. More than 400 mL of fluid must be in the pericardium to lead to a detectable change on plain x-ray. If it is chronic then there may be little functional impairment. An echocardiogram is indicated to detect impairment in right ventricular diastolic filling and to guide drainage.

Abnormalities of the hila and pulmonary vessels

Enlarged hila could be due to an abnormality in any of the three structures that lie there:
- The pulmonary artery (e.g. pulmonary hypertension or pulmonary embolus)
- The main bronchus (e.g. carcinoma)
- Enlarged lymph nodes (e.g. sarcoidosis).

Pulmonary embolism (PE)

Most chest x-rays in patients with a PE are normal (Box 2.2). The primary purpose of a chest film in suspected PE is therefore to rule out other diagnoses as a cause of dysponea or hypoxia. Further imaging is indicated, such as V/Q scan, pulmonary arteriogram and CT pulmonary angiogram (CTPA).

Pleural abnormalities

Pleural effusion

On an upright film, an effusion will cause blunting of the costophrenic angle. Sometimes a depression of the involved diaphragm will occur. A large effusion can lead to a mediastinal

---

Box 2.2 **Chest x-ray signs of pulmonary embolus may include:**
- Westermark's sign (oligemia in affected area)
- Enlarged hilum (caused by thrombus impaction)
- Atelectasis with elevation of hemidiaphragm
- Pleural effusion
- Consolidation

shift. Approximately 200 mL of fluid is needed to detect an effusion in the frontal film – a lateral chest x-ray (though now rarely done) is more sensitive.

In the supine film, an effusion will appear as a graded haze that is denser at the base. To differentiate it from lung disease, vascular shadows can usually be seen through the effusion.

Common causes for a pleural effusion include:
- Congestive heart failure
- Infection (parapneumonic)
- Trauma
- PE
- Tumour
- Autoimmune disease.

Pneumothorax

A pneumothorax is air inside the thoracic cavity but outside the lung. It appears as air without lung markings in the least dependent part of the chest. It is best demonstrated by an expiration film. It can be difficult to see when the patient is in a supine position – air rises to the medial aspect of the lung becoming a lucency along the mediastinum. It may also collect in the inferior sulci causing a deep sulcus sign (Fig. 2.3).

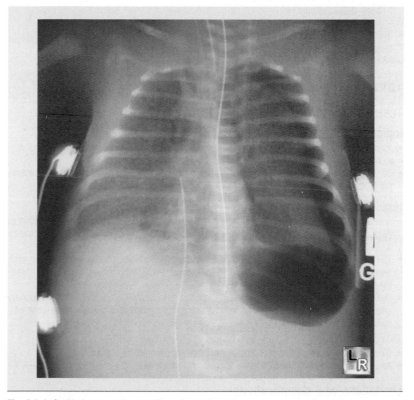

Fig. 2.3 Left-sided pneumothorax with a deep sulcus sign.

Causes of spontaneous pneumothorax include:
- Idiopathic
- Asthma
- COPD
- Pulmonary infection
- Neoplasm
- Marfan syndrome.

A *hydropneumothorax* is both air and fluid in the pleural space. It is characterized by an air–fluid level on an upright or decubitus film in a patient with a pneumothorax.

Further investigations
Computed tomography (CT) scan, ventilation/perfusion (VQ) scan, etc (see below).

Limitations and complications
- To be adequate, a chest x-ray must be:
  - Taken on inspiration (unless suspecting a pneumothorax) – on good inspiration the diaphragm should be at the 8th to 9th posterior rib or the 5th to 6th anterior rib
  - Adequately penetrated – thoracic disc spaces should be visible through the heart but bony details should not
  - Not rotated – medial heads of the clavicles equidistant from vertebral bodies.
- Ionizing radiation is relatively contraindicated for women who might be pregnant. See below for radiation doses.

Other imaging

Test: Computed tomography (CT) scan (Fig. 2.4)

Indications
- Identification of structural thoracic pathologies, including abnormalities of the pulmonary vasculature, lung parenchyma and mediastinum.
- CT pulmonary angiogram (CTPA) is the investigation of choice for diagnosis of nonmassive pulmonary embolus.

How it is done
- A beam of x-rays is passed through the chest and picked up on iodide crystals within a detector. These iodide crystals emit photons when struck by x-rays, which are detected by a photomultiplier.
- The x-ray tube passes around the patient, allowing multiple data to be collected for each section of the chest being viewed. This data is converted by a computer into two- or three-dimensional images.
- Computed tomography can be given with intravenous contrast to highlight the pulmonary arterial tree. This is a CTPA. It can only show central emboli and gives a large dose of radiation to the patient.

Data presented as
- CT scans are viewed 'from the feet up' with the patient on their back.
- As with a conventional x-ray, denser tissues are paler.

Limitations and complications
- CT scans give large doses of radiation to the patient (Box 2.3).

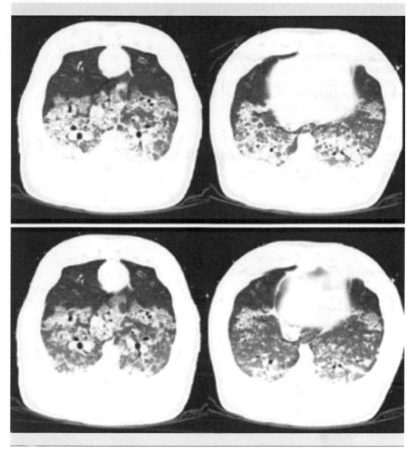

Fig. 2.4 A CT scan consistent with acute lung injury.

Box 2.3 **Radiation dose (millisieverts)**	
Annual background	2.5–3
Chest x-ray	0.1
Abdominal x-ray	2
CT head	2
CT chest	8
CT abdomen	10

- The CT scanner is often in a distant part of the hospital and considerable logistic difficulties arise when transporting a critically ill patient there.
- Medical staff may receive a radiation dose if a patient cannot be left alone in the CT scanner.
- Visualization of the pulmonary vasculature requires intravenous contrast, which is contraindicated in patients with iodine allergy and may worsen renal impairment, especially in patients taking metformin.
- Lesions less than 1 cm in size may be missed.
- CT scans without contrast cannot differentiate between structures of very similar density.

Test: Ventilation-perfusion scan (VQ scan) (Fig. 2.5)

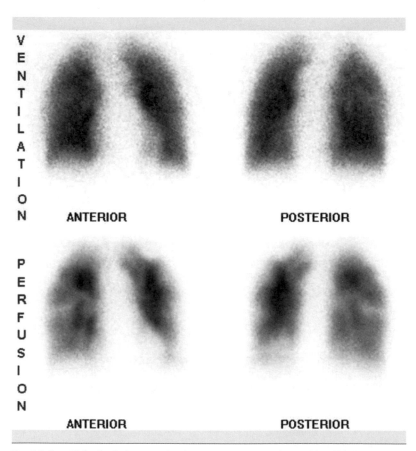

Fig. 2.5 A ventilation/perfusion scan showing multiple perfusion abnormalities. This is suggestive of several pulmonary emboli.

Indications

- Aims to detect mismatches in lung ventilation and perfusion, such as PE.
- Although CTPA is the tool of choice for detection of PE, there is a lower radiation dose for VQ scans than for CTPA, making it the investigation of choice for the pregnant patient with suspected pulmonary embolus.

How it is done

- The pulmonary arterial circulation is viewed using intravenous technetium-99, which fixes in the distal pulmonary capillaries showing where blood is flowing. At the same time, the patient breathes a radioactive gas, usually krypton-81, which shows ventilation in the lungs.

Interpretation

Normal range
- A normal scan shows the same appearance in both the ventilation and perfusion images, showing no mismatch.

Abnormalities
- A PE obstructs distal blood flow and so there are defects in perfusion. This is seen on a ventilation-perfusion scan as a perfusion mismatch, there being no obstruction to ventilation.

Further investigations

- A CTPA may help with diagnosis if the VQ scan is equivocal.

Limitations and complications

- A VQ scan may suffer from poor specificity: any abnormality in lung tissue will affect ventilation and perfusion to some extent. A VQ scan will therefore only detect PE in otherwise fairly normal lungs.
- This investigation exposes the patient to a dose of ionizing radiation, albeit small.
- This investigation cannot usually be done out of hours.

Test: Positron emission tomography (PET) scan

Indications

- Detection of tumours and bony deposits.

How it is done

- PET uses deoxyglucose, a glucose analogue labelled with fluorine-18, which is taken up avidly by malignant cells. Fluorine-18 emits positrons, which combine with electrons to produce photons.

Further investigations

- Staging investigations and tissue diagnosis directs subsequent management.

Limitations and complications

- The (albeit small) dose of radiation given makes this examination relatively contraindicated in pregnant women.
- Because of its reliance on normal glucose metabolism, a PET scan can be unreliable in diabetic patients or those with insulin abnormalities.

Thoracic imaging modality in the trauma patient

Chest CT scans are more sensitive than CXRs for the detection of injuries such as pneumothoraces and pulmonary contusions. Spiral CT has excellent accuracy in this setting but may be suboptimal in assessing arch vessels, where angiography may be more appropriate. Aortic angiography provides images of the entire thoracic aorta and arch vessels that are easy to interpret, however it is a time-consuming technique and availability of service may limit its clinical utility.

More recently increasing use of portable ultrasound devices has allowed early diagnosis of pericardial effusions, and hemothoraces in the emergency department (Focused Assessment with Sonography for Trauma; FAST). The decision to proceed to definitive radiological investigation is always a balance of risk versus benefit in the trauma setting. Full ATLS patient assessment and treatment is mandated prior to transfer.

Pulmonary function tests

Test: Functional residual capacity (FRC; Fig. 2.6)

Indications

• Although measured infrequently, it is an important physiological concept for anaesthetists.

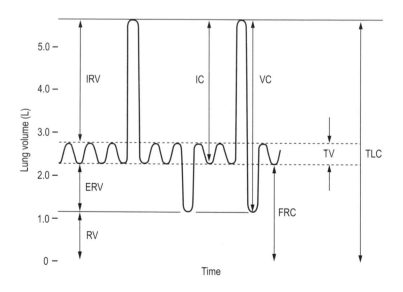

Fig. 2.6 Normal spirometry. ERV, expiratory reserve volume; FRC, functional residual capacity; IC, inspiratory capacity; IRV, inspiratory reserve volume; RV, residual volume; VC, vital capacity; TLC, total lung capacity.

How FRC is measured
- Steady-state or single breath helium dilution, nitrogen washout or whole body plethysmography.
- Steady-state helium dilution involves connecting the patient to a helium-containing spirometer at the end of a normal exhalation: the change in helium concentration allows a calculation of FRC.

Interpretation
Normal value
20 mL/kg approximately 1.5 L in a 70-kg adult male.

Physiological principles
FRC is:
- The combination of residual volume and expiratory reserve volume
- The volume left in the lungs after a normal exhalation
- The lung volume at elastic equilibrium
- Tested in combination with other lung volumes
- Important as during apnoea it is an oxygen reservoir: if it falls below closing capacity, airway closure (and potential hypoxia) will occur during tidal breathing.

Abnormalities
Reduced
- Restrictive lung disease (e.g. pulmonary fibrosis).
- Extrinsic lung compression (e.g. obesity, plural effusion, scoliosis).
- Reduced lung volume (e.g. post pneumonectomy).
- Pregnancy, lying supine, neonates.
- Neuromuscular disease (e.g. Guillain-Barré syndrome).

Increased
- Airflow obstruction: emphysema, asthma.
- The elderly patient.

Further investigations
- Flow/volume curves and arterial blood gas analysis.

Limitations and complications
- Dependent on age, sex and height.

Test: Volume/time curve (Fig. 2.7)

Indications
With flow/volume curves, occasionally used preoperatively to:
- Investigate cause of shortness of breath (to differentiate obstructive from restrictive lung disease)
- Assess degree of disease
- Assess response to treatment (e.g. pre/post β_2 agonist) and decide if treatment is 'optimal'.

How it is done
- Measured by spirometer, which alone cannot measure volumes that do not take part in normal ventilation (i.e. residual volume (RV) and FRC).
- Subject takes a full breath in and blows out as long, hard and completely as possible then takes a full breath in before resuming normal breathing.
- Repeated three times to ensure acceptable and reproducible results.

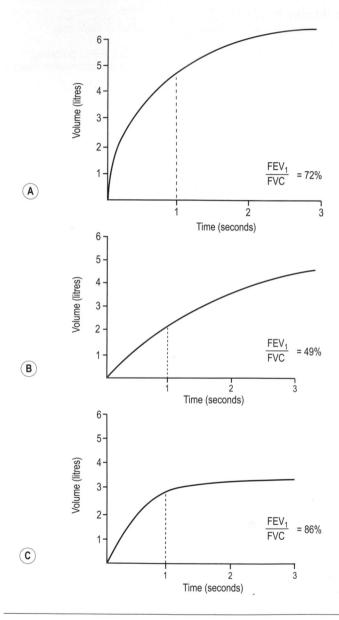

Fig. 2.7 Volume/time curves: (A) normal; (B) obstructive; (C) restrictive.

- Volume/times are recorded and compared to predicted (% expected).
- Volume exhaled in 1 second (FEV_1) is compared to the volume of all that can be maximally forcefully exhaled (FVC, forced vital capacity), giving a ratio.
- Results may be compared before/after bronchodilators ('reversibility').

Interpretation

Data presented as graphs and numerical data (absolute numbers, % predicted).

Normal range/graph
- Normal FEV_1/FVC = 70–80%.

Abnormalities

Obstructive lung defect: FEV_1/FVC = <70%
- The volume expired in 1 second is disproportionately small and the volume/time curve is flatter.
- Example: COPD, asthma.

Restrictive lung defect: FEV_1/FVC = >80%
- Due to smaller total lung volume.
- Example: lung fibrosis, chest wall disease.

Further investigations
- Flow/volume curves and peak expiratory flow rate (PEFR) are usually measured at the same time.

Limitations and complications
- Technique, recent use of bronchodilators, exercise, age, height, gender and ethnicity can all affect results.

Test: Flow/volume curve (dynamic)

Indications
- See volume/time curves.

How it is done
- Principle similar to volume-time curves.
- Results may be compared before/after bronchodilators ('reversibility').
- PEFR, peak inspiratory flow rate (PIFR), FVC may also be measured.

Interpretation

Data presented as graphs and numerical data (absolute numbers, % predicted).

Normal range/graph
- Normal: Fig. 2.8A.

Abnormalities
- Intrathoracic airway obstruction
  - Airway compression during expiration produces a characteristic 'curvilinear' shape (Fig. 2.8B)
  - Increasingly severe disease lowers PEFR and FVC
  - Common causes: emphysema/bronchitis; asthma; bronchiectasis.
- Extrathoracic obstruction (Fig. 2.9).

A fixed obstruction reduces both peak expiratory and inspiratory flow rates
  - On expiration, extrathoracic airway pressures are above atmospheric and hold the airway open: expiration is less affected

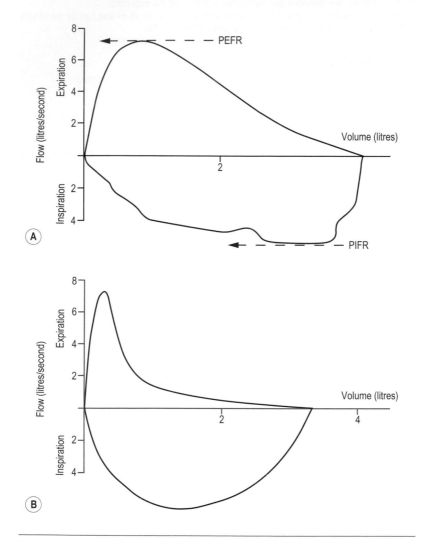

Fig. 2.8 Flow-volume loops in (A) normal and (B) mild intrathoracic airway obstruction.

– On inspiration, the decreased extrathoracic airway pressures narrow the airway, hence a greater effect on inspiration
– Causes include: tracheal stenosis, laryngeal paralysis, goitre.

A variable obstruction may be held open during expiration by the above atmospheric extrathoracic airway pressures, so expiration is relatively unaffected.

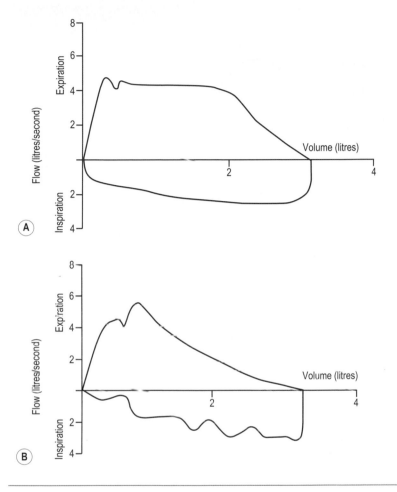

Fig. 2.9 Flow-volume loops in (A) fixed and (B) variable extrathoracic obstruction.

Causes include pharyngeal muscle weakness of Obstructive Sleep Apnoea, laryngeal tumour
• Respiratory muscle weakness (Fig. 2.10). Lower pressure/slower rise of airway pressures cause:
    – Lower, later PEFR in expiration and lower flow throughout inspiration
    – Loss of large airway flow changes ('expiratory spikes') when the patient is asked to cough (a test rarely done clinically).
Restrictive lung disease
    – Reduced Vital capacity, PEFR and accelerated emptying.

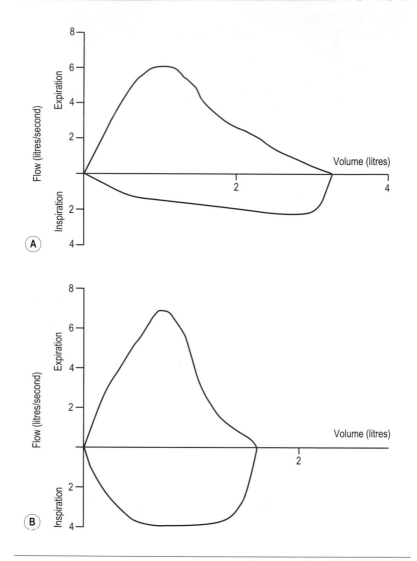

Fig. 2.10 Flow-volume loop in (A) respiratory muscle weakness and (B) restrictive disease.

Further investigations

- Volume/time curves (generating FEV_1/FVC) are usually measured.

Limitations and complications

- See volume/time curves.

Test: Transfer factor/diffusing capacity

Indications

- To investigate disorders of the alveolar membrane.

How it is done

- 0.03% carbon monoxide (CO) along with 10% helium (to measure alveolar volume) is held in a single breath for 10 seconds: the expired gas concentrations are measured.
- If the subject is normal, then CO will be able to diffuse across the alveolus and the exhaled CO concentration will be appropriately low, resulting in a normal transfer factor.
- The results are based on three factors:
  1. The properties/surface area of the alveolar-capillary membrane
  2. The binding of CO to haemoglobin
  3. The amount of haemoglobin in pulmonary microcirculation.
- The result may be expressed as a transfer factor or as a transfer coefficient per volume lung, K_{CO} (mmol/min/kPa/L).
- K_{CO} helps differentiate conditions in which there is a reduction in surface area that is normal (e.g. pneumonectomy) from those where the surface area may be reduced, but there is abnormal alveolar membrane (e.g. emphysema).

Interpretation

Normal value

Normal T_{LCO} = 10–15 mmol/min/kPa in a 25-year-old male.

Abnormalities

- Reduced T_{LCO} but normal K_{CO}: reduced lung volume with normal remaining gas transfer: $\downarrow$ effort or respiratory muscle weakness, thoracic deformity, lung resection, anaemia.
- Reduced T_{LCO} but low K_{CO}: reduced lung volume with abnormal gas transfer: emphysema, pulmonary emboli, interstitial lung disease (e.g. pulmonary fibrosis, sarcoidosis), pulmonary hypertension, pulmonary vasculitis, pulmonary oedema, excess carboxyhaemoglobin, pregnancy (12–26 weeks).
- Increased T_{LCO}: polycythaemia, left-to-right shunt, pulmonary haemorrhage, asthma, exercise, pregnancy (up to 12 weeks).

Further investigations

- Performed with measurement of lung volumes, flow/volume curves and arterial blood gas.

Limitations and complications

- Dependent on age, sex and height.
- Subjects must not have recently exercised, smoked, be anaemic or polycythaemic.

Intraoperative respiratory monitoring

Test: Pulse oximetry (SpO$_2$)

Indications
Pulse oximetry is a minimum monitoring standard for anyone undergoing anaesthesia or sedation. It is used in recovery, any high dependency or intensive care situation, anyone with respiratory or cardiovascular compromise, or any patient considered likely to deteriorate. Pulse oximeters also measure pulse rate and estimate pulse regularity; thus they are used as an intermittent observation for any hospital inpatient. It is also used after plastic or orthopaedic surgery distal to the affected site, as a surrogate marker of perfusion.

Physiological principles
Oxyhaemoglobin absorbs different light wavelengths compared to deoxyhaemoglobin. The wavelength of light absorbed corresponds to the degree of oxygenation of the haemoglobin.

How it is done
A source of light comes from a probe (on the finger or ear) at two wavelengths (usually 650 nm and 805 nm). The light is partially absorbed by haemoglobin, by amounts which differ depending on how much saturated with oxygen it is. By calculating the absorption at the two wavelengths, a processor can display the proportion of haemoglobin that is oxygenated. The processor subtracts the non-pulsatile part, leaving only the arterial component.

Interpretation
Oxygen saturation is expressed as a percentage of oxygen *content* of haemoglobin, as a proportion of oxygen *capacity* of haemoglobin. Normal ranges are 97–100% for a healthy subject breathing room air. Any form of cardiac or respiratory disease may reduce it.

Management principles
A low SpO$_2$ in the absence of artefact indicates that the oxygen saturation of arterial blood is poor. This should be corrected depending upon the underlying cause; increasing the fractional inspired oxygen concentration (FiO$_2$) may be helpful in the absence of shunt.

Limitations and complications
Pulse oximetry is subject to inaccuracies. Artefact may be caused by flickering overhead lights, shivering, poor arterial pulsation, certain nail varnishes or inks, and the presence of carbon monoxide (carboxyhaemoglobin tends towards an oximeter reading of 100%) and methaemoglobinaemia (tends towards 85%). A venous pulsation due to tricuspid regurgitation will cause low readings.

Oxygen saturation is not a marker of ventilation, especially if supplemental oxygen is being administered. Similarly, one cannot comment on oxygen delivery to the tissues, which is also affected by haemoglobin concentration and cardiac output. Because the calibration is carried out on healthy volunteers, readings below 70% are inaccurate.

Test: Capnography

Indications
A requirement of minimum monitoring standards for patients undergoing general anaesthesia. It gives useful information on:
- CO$_2$ production and removal
- Lung perfusion

- Alveolar ventilation
- Altered airway dynamics
- Respiratory pattern and adverse respiratory events.

How it is done

Most commonly measured by infrared (IR) spectography. Expired CO_2 is a polyatomic gas and absorbs IR rays (specific wavelengths around 4.8 μm).

Interpretation

The amount absorbed is proportional to the concentration of the absorbing gas present. Concentration of CO_2 can be determined by comparing the measured absorbance with the absorbance of a known standard.

Data presented as

End tidal CO_2 ($P_{ET}CO_2$), expressed as partial pressure, measured in kPa or mmHg.

Physiological principles

During the respiratory cycle exhaled CO_2 produces a display of instantaneous CO_2 concentration versus time. In the healthy patient, end-tidal CO_2 ($P_{ET}CO_2$) closely approximates to arterial CO_2 ($PaCO_2$). CO_2 in exhaled gas is dependent on its carriage from site of production in the tissues to the lungs via the right heart (Table 2.1). Thus capnography also provides limited but useful information on cardiac output, pulmonary blood flow and the diffusion of pulmonary capillary gases. A mismatch between $P_{ET}CO_2$ and $PaCO_2$ may occur due to both physiological and pathological processes.

Table 2.1 Conditions affecting arterial – end-tidal CO_2 gradient	
Increasing gradient	**Decreasing gradient**
Age	Increased cardiac output
COPD	Low frequency ventilation
Pulmonary embolism	Pregnancy
Reduced cardiac output	Infants under anaesthesia
Hypovolaemia	
General anaesthesia	

Normal range

In the healthy patient $P_{ET}CO_2$ approximates $PaCO_2$ (5–5.6 kPa). Figure 2.11 shows four phases of a normal capnograph trace:

Phase 1 – baseline trace should read zero when no re-breathing occurs

Phase 2 – upstroke as exhaled dead space gas mixes with alveolar gas

Phase 3 – plateau represents alveolar CO_2 mixing

Phase 4 – inspiration occurs and CO_2 falls to zero.

Abnormalities and management principles

See Fig. 2.12.

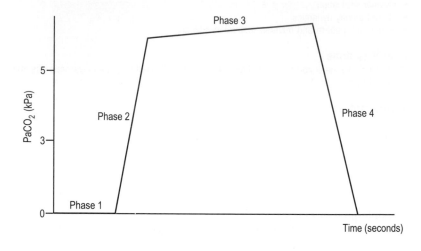

Fig. 2.11 Four phases of a normal capnograph trace.

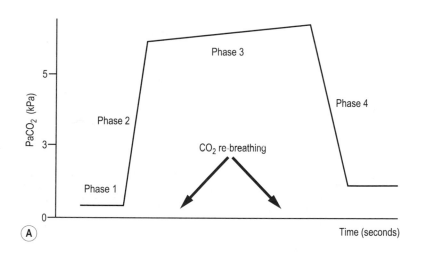

Fig. 2.12 (A) Baseline elevated suggests CO_2 re-breathing. Check anaesthetic circuitry and gas flow rate.

(Continued)

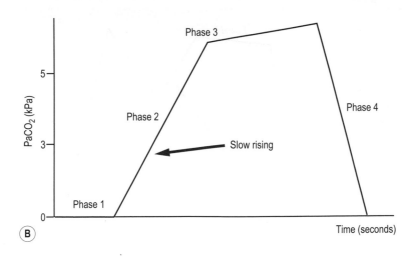

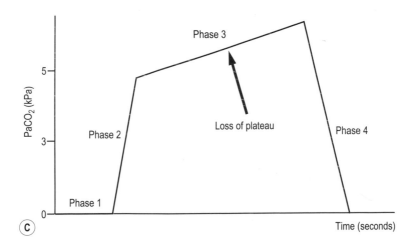

Fig. 2.12 cont'd. (B) Slow upstroke phase 2 suggests obstruction to expiratory gas flow (e.g. asthma, bronchospasm, COPD and kinked endotracheal tube or in the presence of leaks in the breathing system). Examine patient and anaesthetic circuit. (C) Loss of plateau in phase 3 suggests differing time constants in the lung seen with COPD and emphysema. Examine and optimize patient treatment.

(Continued)

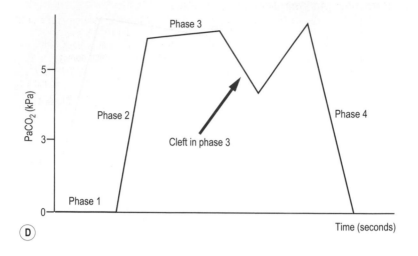

Fig. 2.12 cont'd. (D) Cleft signifies return of respiratory effort during mechanical ventilation or artefact associated with abdominal movement during surgery. Check adequacy of muscle paralysis.

Test: Shunt fraction

Indications
Hypoxaemia may be the result of shunting. Understanding its basis allows a rational approach to its correction.

How it is done
The total physiological shunt fraction can be calculated using the shunt equation, which allows calculation of the amount of venous blood bypassing ventilated alveoli and mixing with pulmonary end-capillary blood:

$$\frac{Q_s}{Q_t} = \frac{(CcO_2 - CaO_2)}{(CcO_2 - CvO_2)}$$

where CcO_2 = end-capillary O_2 content, CaO_2 = arterial O_2 content and CvO_2 = mixed venous O_2 content.

Physiological principles
When blood flow and oxygen content is known, the amount of shunt flow and its impact on systemic arterial oxygenation can be calculated. The shunt is described as a percentage of the cardiac output. Anatomical shunt exists with normal anatomy, e.g. thebesian and bronchial veins contribute a small degree of shunt in all humans by emptying into the left heart.

Abnormal anatomical shunts are best divided into pulmonary and/or extrapulmonary, e.g. pulmonary arteriovenous fistula or an atrial septal defect:

Physiological shunt = VQ inequalities + anatomical shunt

Abnormalities and management principles

In clinical practice a degree of shunting may be seen due to altered VQ matching associated with anaesthetic agent use, intermittent positive pressure ventilation (IPPV), patient positioning and hydration status. However, shunt is commonly the result of pulmonary pathology including pneumonia, atelectasis and pulmonary oedema, which during anaesthesia may prove difficult to treat. True shunts respond poorly to increased oxygen concentration, but improvement in oxygenation may be seen with attention to the conduct of anaesthesia and optimizing cardiac output, ventilatory settings including positive end expiratory pressure (PEEP) and patient positioning, thus correcting VQ inequalities.

Further investigations

Shunt estimation 1: Alveolar–arterial gradient (A-a gradient)

The degree of shunt can be estimated by comparing the partial pressure of O_2 in the alveoli (A) to that in the artery (a). The A-a gradient is ($PAO_2 - PaO_2$)

$$PAO_2 = (\text{barometric pressure} - \text{saturated water vapour pressure}) \times FO_2$$
$$- PaCO_2/\text{respiratory quotient}$$

$$PAO_2 = (101 - 6.3) \times FiO_2 - PaCO_2/0.8 \text{ (or 1)}$$

This is the alveolar gas equation.

A normal A-a gradient is approximately 20 in a healthy young person and a rough estimation is (age + 10)/4 (mmHg). A-a increases 5–7 mmHg for every 10% increase in FiO_2.

Shunt estimation 2: Arterial/alveolar ratio (a/A ratio)

Here the same values as for the A-a gradient are divided rather than subtracted (PaO_2/PAO_2). Further simplification by substituting PAO_2 for FiO_2 offers a rough but useful estimate of shunt for clinical practice.

Shunt estimation 3: 'P/F' ratio (PaO_2/FiO_2)

This compares the arterial oxygen tension with the fractional inspired oxygen concentration and has the advantage of not using the alveolar gas equation (Table 2.2).

Table 2.2 **Example of shunt estimation P/F**		
PaO_2 kPa (mmHg)	**FiO_2**	**P/F ratio**
12.5 (93.7)	0.21	59 (446)
10 (75)	0.30	33 (250)
8 (60)	0.70	11 (86)

Pressure–volume (P/V) curve analysis

Test: Static airway compliance

Data presented as

Compliance is defined as the volume change per unit pressure change ($\Delta V/\Delta P$) (mL/cmH$_2$O), a measure of lung distensibility.

Physiological principles

Many diseases result in altered pulmonary elasticity, which can be measured by changes in compliance ($\Delta V/\Delta P$), or elastance ($\Delta P/\Delta V$).

During spontaneous ventilation the total compliance of the chest wall and lungs is approximately 100 mL/cmH$_2$0. The lung compliance is approximately 200 mL/cmH$_2$0. During ventilated anaesthesia, total compliance of the respiratory system is approximately 70–80 mL/cmH$_2$0.

Indications for measurement

1. A research tool to analyze the mechanical properties of the respiratory system.
2. To guide ventilatory adjustments to optimize mechanical ventilation.
3. As a limited model to appreciate lung protective ventilation strategies.

How it is done

1. The inspiratory occlusion technique involves the sequential measurement of plateau airway pressures corresponding to different tidal volumes during successive end inspiratory occlusions.
   - In the paralyzed patient
   - Sequentially inflating the lungs with a known volume of gas and measuring the transmural pressure (between atmosphere and airway pressure when there is no airflow)
2. The quasi-static method uses a continuous inflation at a constant gas flow. Here the change in airway pressure is inversely proportional to the compliance of the respiratory system. A simple technique, the graphic is often incorporated into ventilator screen settings.

Interpretation

The lung at residual volume requires an opening pressure before inflation takes place. A lower inflection point indicates the pressure at which many collapsed alveoli are opening at the same time. Application of PEEP that is equal to or greater than the pressure corresponding to the lower inflection point results in significant alveolar recruitment and decrease in pulmonary shunt. This approach may avoid mechanical ventilation-induced lung injury resulting from the repeated opening and closure of the terminal bronchioles during each respiratory cycle.

The P-V relationship is linear around FRC until total lung capacity (TLC) is approached as denoted by an upper inflection point (UIP) (Fig. 2.13). Above UIP overdistension of alveolar units occurs and no more recruitment is achieved. On the P/V curve this point is situated around 30 cmH$_2$0. A stiff lung (e.g. ARDS) has a low compliance, whereas a highly distensible lung (e.g. emphysema) has a high compliance.

Compliance is affected by posture, and will be increased with age and emphysematous lung disease. Increases in extravascular lung water, consolidation, poorly adjusted mechanical ventilation and fibrosis are common causes of reduced compliance.

Limitations of technique

May require a patient to be paralyzed and disconnected from the ventilator. Inspiratory hold techniques are also time consuming and may be subject to error when intrinsic PEEP is present. The quasi-static technique may be of limited use where high gas flow rates result in high airway resistance as a source of error.

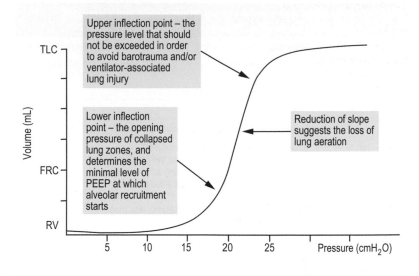

Fig. 2.13 Pressure–volume curve used to measure compliance. FRC, functional residual capacity; RV, residual volume; TLC, total lung capacity.

Blood gas analysis

Test: Arterial blood gas analysis

Indications
- To diagnose acid-base disorders and monitor treatment.
- To assess adequacy of ventilation and oxygenation.

How it is done
- Anticoagulated blood from an arterial line or arterial puncture is used.
- Electrodes measure the pH, PO_2 (Clark) and PCO_2 (Severinghaus).
- The bicarbonate, base excess/deficit is calculated.
- Some machines may also measure haemoglobin photometrically as well as electrolytes and lactate.
- Co-oximeters haemolyze the blood and measure total haemoglobin, fetal haemoglobin, oxyhaemoglobin, deoxyhaemoglobin, carboxyhaemoglobin and methaemoglobin by using absorbance at six different wavelengths, which is more accurate than photometric methods.

Interpretation
See Table 2.3.

Physiological principles
- Disorders may be classified according to the pH (acidaemia or alkalaemia) and whether the cause is respiratory (CO_2) or metabolic (bicarbonate).
- Each disorder may be compensated (tending to normalize the pH) or mixed (a combined metabolic/respiratory disorder).
- Acidosis is a tendency to acidaemia and alkalosis is a tendency to alkalaemia.

Table 2.3 **Definitions and normal ranges of measured and calculated acid-base parameters breathing room air at sea level**

Abbreviation	Meaning	Normal value
pH	A measurement of the hydrogen ion concentration (log scale) $pH = pK + log\ ([HCO_3^-]/[CO_2])$	7.35–7.45
PCO_2	Partial pressure of CO_2	4.8–5.9 kPa
PO_2	Partial pressure of O_2; the FiO_2 must be known	11.9–13.2 kPa
BEx	Base excess, a measure of the metabolic component of acid-base disorders: the calculated amount in milliequivalents of strong acid required to restore 1 litre of fully saturated blood to pH 7.4, at a PCO_2 of 5.3 kPa More than +2 = a metabolic alkalosis; less than −2 = a metabolic acidosis	−2 to +2
sBEx	Standard base excess: the calculated base excess after the sample has been equilibrated ('standardized') with CO_2 at 5.3 kPa at 37°C, saturated with oxygen and a haemoglobin of 5 g/dL	−2 to +2
BDef	Base deficit: a measure of the metabolic component of acid-base disorders; is the opposite of base excess	−2 to +2
Total CO_2	$= CO_2 + HCO_3^-$	22–32 mEq/L
$sHCO_3$	Standard bicarbonate: the calculated bicarbonate concentration after the sample has been equilibrated ('standardized') with CO_2 at 5.3 kPa at 37°C and saturated with oxygen. Like base excess, a measure of the purely metabolic component	22–26 mmol/L
$aHCO_3$	Actual bicarbonate: the bicarbonate calculated from the measured CO_2 and pH; values vary if the CO_2 is abnormal	22–26 mmol/L

Abnormalities
- The disorder can be calculated by working through Fig. 2.14 (below).
- Respiratory compensation for metabolic disorder: the minute volume will change in minutes to alter CO_2.
- Metabolic compensation for a respiratory disorder: renal bicarbonate reabsorption will change within 12 hours, but complete correction takes some days.

Low pH with low $sHCO_3$ (<22) or BEx (<−2.2): Metabolic acidosis
- Acid ingestion, e.g. aspirin overdose.
- ↑ Acid production
  - Lactic acidosis type A and B, e.g. hypovolaemia, sepsis, cardiac failure – see topic 9 for more details of lactic acidosis
  - Diabetic Ketoacidosis: β hydroxybutyrate and acetoacetate
  - Hyperchloraemia – excess saline-containing fluids (e.g. most colloids) especially with hypernatraemia
  - Hepatic failure

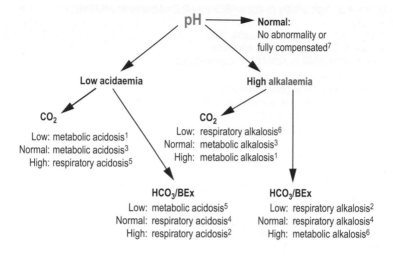

Fig. 2.14 Flow diagram for interpretation of acid-base abnormalities. [1]with attempted respiratory compensation (either acute or chronic); [2]with attempted metabolic compensation (i.e. treated with bicarbonate or longer than ~ 6 hours); [3]with no respiratory compensation; [4]with no metabolic compensation; [5]mixed respiratory/metabolic acidosis if CO_2 high *and* HCO_3/BEx low; [6]mixed respiratory/metabolic alkalosis if CO_2 low *and* HCO_3/BEx high; [7]acid-base disturbances are rarely fully compensated by the patient's natural mechanisms.

- Glucose-6-phosphate dehydrogenase deficiency
- Drugs: metformin, alcohols, reverse transcriptase inhibitors
- Thiamine deficiency.
- ↓ Acid elimination
  - Renal failure: organic acids, e.g. sulphuric acid
  - Distal renal tubular acidosis.
- ↑ Bicarbonate loss
  - Diarrhoea, large ileostomy losses, small bowel fistulae
  - Urethroenterostomy, proximal renal tubular acidosis.

Low pH with high pCO_2 (>6.2 kPa): Respiratory acidosis
Chronic hypoventilation is compensated by HCO_3 retention.
- Acute hypoventilation
  - Central control – e.g. CNS depressant drugs, fatigue, CO_2 narcosis, encephalitis, brainstem disease, trauma
  - Airway obstruction – large (e.g. blocked cuffed oral endotracheal tube, COETT) or small airways (e.g. bronchitis/emphysema)
  - Respiratory muscle weakness or paralysis
  - Reduced lung volume – e.g. pneumonia, reduced artificial ventilation, structural chest abnormalities
- Excess CO_2 production/administration
  - Hypermetabolism (e.g. malignant hyperthermia)
  - Failure of CO_2 absorber – re-breathing
  - Iatrogenic CO_2 administration.

High pH with high sHCO$_3$ (>26) or BEx (>+2.2): Metabolic alkalosis
- ↑ Acid loss
  - Prolonged vomiting/loss of gastric fluid
  - Conn's, Cushing's, Bartter's syndrome.
- ↑ Base administration, retention or concentration
  - Excess bicarbonate
  - Excess citrate (e.g. blood transfusion)
  - Excess buffer in renal haemofiltration fluid (e.g. lactate)
  - Loss of Cl$^-$ (e.g. diuretics)
  - Renal retention of bicarbonate.

High pH with low pCO$_2$ (<4.2 kPa): Respiratory alkalosis
This is caused by hyperventilation.
- Excess external mechanical ventilation.
- Central nervous system: pain, anxiety, fever, cerebrovascular accident, systemic inflammatory response, meningitis, encephalitis.
- Hypoxaemia: high altitude, severe anaemia, right-to-left shunts.
- Drugs: e.g. doxapram, aminophyline, salicylate, catecholamines, stimulants.
- Endocrine: pregnancy and hyperthyroidism.
- Stimulation of chest receptors.
- pneumothorax/haemothorax, pulmonary infection/oedema/aspiration/embolism, interstitial lung disease.

Management principles
- Identify and treat the cause.
- Intravenous sodium bicarbonate (8.4% 50 mL/hour) may worsen intracellular acidosis, but may buy time if there is a rapid rise in serum K$^+$, the acidosis is severe (e.g. pH <7.1) or if definitive treatment is awaited.

Further investigations
- Anion gap $= ([Na^+] + [K^+]) - ([Cl^-] + [HCO_3^-])$

Strictly, it refers to the venous electrolyte concentrations.

In the context of a metabolic acidosis:
- 8–16 mEq/L = renal/GI HCO$_3^-$ losses, or ↓ renal acid excretion
- >16 mEq/L = an unmeasured anion, e.g. lactic, methanol, ethanol, ketoacids, paraldehyde, renal failure, etc (See Intensive Care topic for more information)
- <8 mEq/L = hyponatraemia, hypoalbuminaemia, paraproteinaemia
- Strong ion difference = the difference in concentration between strong cations and strong anions:

  Normal $- \sim 40mEq/L$
  $$= [Na^+] + [K^+] + [Ca^{2+}] + [Mg^{2+}] - [Cl^-] - [\text{Other strong anions}]$$

  - A. strong ion is a highly dissociated cation or anion
  - Concept developed by Peter Stewart (1981)
  - Stewart showed that metabolic changes in acid-base disorders were due to:
    - The strong ion difference or
    - [ATOT], total plasma concentration of the weak nonvolatile acids – inorganic phosphate or serum proteins such as albumin.

Limitations and complications
- Heparin (an acid) lowers the pH: expel the heparin before taking the sample.
- Large air bubble in the syringe may raise pO$_2$ and pH and lower pCO$_2$: expel the air.
- Abnormal plasma protein levels affect the base excess/bicarbonate.
- Intravenous lipid may affect pH.

TOPIC ❸

Cardiovascular system

Topic Contents

Perioperative cardiac risk
assessment 37
Test: Risk assessment scoring 37
Test: Cardiopulmonary Exercise Testing
(CPEX) 39
Test: Electrocardiogram (ECG) 41
Test: Exercise tolerance test (ETT) 47
Test: Biochemical markers of myocardial
ischaemia 47
Echocardiography 49
Test: Transthoracic echocardiography
(TTE) and transoesophageal
echocardiography (TOE) 49

Cardiac catheterization 52
Test: Coronary angiography 52
Test: Right heart catheterization 53
Test: Cardiac tomography angiogram
(CTA) 54
Nuclear imaging 55
Test: Thallium/technetium scan 55
Test: Technetium-99-labelled sestamibi 56
Test: Cardiac MRI (CMR) 56

Perioperative cardiac risk assessment

Indications

- Identify those at significant risk of developing perioperative cardiac complications.
- Prioritize investigation and treatment prior to surgery.

Test: Risk assessment scoring

In 1977 Goldman and colleagues developed a preoperative cardiac risk index (Table 3.1) based on nine clinical factors to give a cumulative risk score, predicting outcome after noncardiac surgery.

In 1986 this was modified by Detsky (Table 3.2) to include angina, suspected aortic valve disease and pulmonary oedema. Based on this model patients are stratified as low, intermediate or high risk for a cardiac event.

The American College of Cardiology (ACC)/American Heart Association (AHA) provide a structured evidence-based approach to perioperative cardiovascular risk evaluation, which incorporates clinical predictors, functional capacity (see below) and surgery-specific risks.

Table 3.1 Goldman risk prediction index

Risk factor	Score	
Third heart sound (S3)	11	**Score >25**
Elevated jugular venous pulse	11	56% risk of death
Myocardial infarct within 6/12 months of surgery	10	22% risk severe CVS complications
Heart rhythm other than sinus rhythm	7	**<25**
ECG with >5 premature ventricular beats	7	4% risk of death 17% risk of severe CVS complications.
Age >70	5	**<6**
Emergency surgery	4	0.2% risk of death 0.7% risk of severe CVS complications
Intrathoracic/intra-abdominal or aortic aneurysm surgery	3	
Poor general health status or bed ridden	3	

Table 3.2 Detsky's modified cardiac risk index

Factor	Risk
Age older than 70 years	5
Myocardial infection within 6 months	10
Myocardial infection after 6 months	5
Canadian Cardiovascular Society Angina Classification*	
Class III	10
Class IV	20
Unstable angina within 6 months	10
Alveolar pulmonary oedema	
Within 1 week	10
Any history of pulmonary oedema	5
Suspected critical aortic stenosis	20
Arrhythmia	
Rhythm other than sinus plus atrial premature beats	5
More than five premature ventricular beats	5
Emergency operation	10
Poor general medical status	5

Class	Points	Cardiac risk
I	0–15	Low
II	20–30	
III	31+	High

*The Canadian Cardiovascular Society Angina Grading Scale is commonly used for the classification of severity of angina: Class I – angina only during strenuous or prolonged physical activity; Class II – slight limitation, with angina only during vigorous physical activity; Class III – symptoms with everyday living activities, i.e., moderate limitation; Class IV – inability to perform any activity without angina or angina at rest, i.e., severe limitation.

Metabolic equivalent task (MET)

METs are a measure of functional capacity, which estimate the energy requirement to carry out activities of daily living (Table 3.3). One MET is defined as the average resting oxygen uptake for a 70-kg male and is equal to approximately 3.5 mL/kg/min. Assessment predicts a patient's exercise capacity, which may contribute to patient risk assessment.

The AHA/ACC guidelines suggest that patients unable to meet a 4-MET demand are at increased perioperative and long-term risk.

Table 3.3 **MET (metabolic equivalent) values**	
No of METs	**Activity**
2 METs	Eat, dress or use the toilet. Walk indoors around the house. Walk on level ground at 2–3 mph or 3.2–4.8 km/h
4 METs	Light work around the house like dusting or washing dishes. Climb a flight of stairs or walk up a hill. Walk on level ground at 4 mph or 6.4 km/h. Participate in moderate recreational activities like golf, bowling
>10 METs	Participate in strenuous sports like swimming, singles tennis, football, basketball or skiing

Adapted from the Duke Activity Status Index and AHA Exercise Standards.

Test: Cardiopulmonary exercise testing (CPEX)

Indications

- Allows a functional capacity assessment of the cardiopulmonary unit and determines its ability to deliver oxygen (DO_2) during exercise.
- Enables identification of high-risk populations who might benefit from invasive monitoring and cardiac optimization to improve DO_2 and surgical outcome.

How it is done

The subject breathes into a mouthpiece whilst exercising on a bicycle or treadmill to a predefined protocol. Total oxygen uptake (VO_2), minute ventilation (VE) and carbon dioxide production (VCO_2) are measured by continuous respiratory gas analysis, as are blood pressure and ECG.

Interpretation

VO_2max (Fig. 3.1): Represents maximal oxygen uptake during exercise of increasing intensity. Expressed in mL/kg/min, VO_2max is a function of both the maximal cardiac output and the maximal tissue extraction of O_2. Under exercise conditions, oxygen consumption becomes a linear function of cardiac output. This measurement is therefore an indirect measure of ventricular function.

Anaerobic threshold (AT) (Figs 3.2 and 3.3): This is the point during exercise at which anaerobic metabolism is used to supplement aerobic metabolism as a source of energy. In exercise, when lactate is produced it is buffered by bicarbonate, leading to increased production of CO_2. This causes a rise in VCO_2, which exceeds the rise in VO_2, therefore the VCO_2/VO_2 ratio increases.

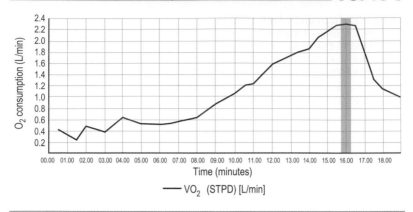

Fig. 3.1 Maximal oxygen uptake (VO$_2$) during exercise of increasing intensity as a measure of ventricular function and oxygen delivery (STPD = standard temperature (0°C), barometric pressure at sea level (101.3 kPa) and dry gas: standard temperature and pressure, dry).

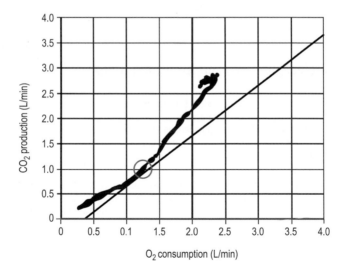

Fig. 3.2 Anaerobic threshold can be measured as the point at which the patient's gas analysis (red line) during exercise fails to track the normal relationship between oxygen consumption and carbon dioxide production during increasing aerobic metabolism (brown line).

An AT of >11 mL/min/kg predicted postoperative survival with a high sensitivity and specificity. Cardiovascular death was virtually confined to patients with an AT <11 mL/min/kg. Older P. Chest 1999. 116(2)355–62

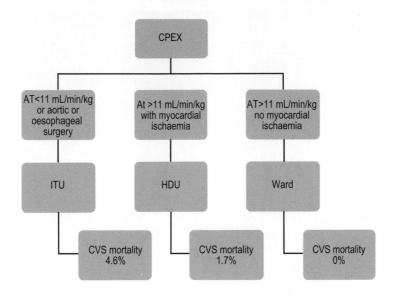

Fig. 3.3 Implications of anaerobic threshold (AT) with respect to perioperative cardiovascular risk. (Adapted from Older P et al. Chest 1999. 116(2) 355–62 Cardiopulmonary exercise testing as a screening test for perioperative management of major surgery in the elderly.)

Test: Electrocardiogram (ECG)

Indication
To assess cardiac rhythm and to identify cardiovascular pathology contributing to surgical risk, e.g. previous infarcts, conduction defects, bundle branch block and strain patterns. National Institute for Clinical Excellence (NICE) guidelines indicate which patients require preoperative ECGs.

How it is done
See Fig. 3.4 for ECG lead placement.

Interpretation
Review morphology of ECG waveforms and complexes (Fig. 3.5)
- The P wave – atrial depolarization.
- The QRS complex – depolarization of the ventricles.
- The ST segment – connects QRS complex and T wave. It starts at the J-point (junction between the QRS complex and ST segment) and ends at the beginning of the T wave.
- T wave – represents repolarization of the ventricles.
- U wave – not always seen but if present represents repolarization of the papillary muscles and purkinje fibres.

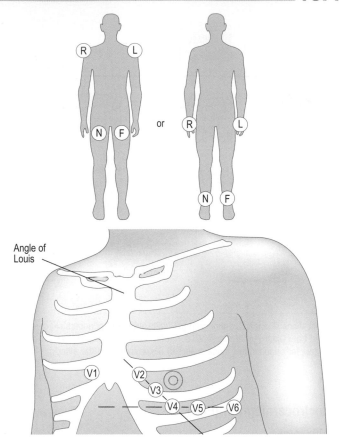

Fig. 3.4 ECG lead placement.

Establish rhythm and conduction pattern
- Look for P waves and their relation to the QRS complex to confirm sinus rhythm. Measure PR interval, QRS complex and QT interval to exclude conduction defects.

Calculate heart rate
- At an ECG paper speed of 25 mm/second each small square is 0.04 seconds.
- The heart rate can be calculated by counting the number of large squares between two consecutive R waves, and dividing this number into 300.

Assess axis
See Table 3.4.
- Look at leads I and aVF – if the predominant (total) QRS deflection (R wave in millimetres minus S wave in millimetres) is a positive value the axis is normal.

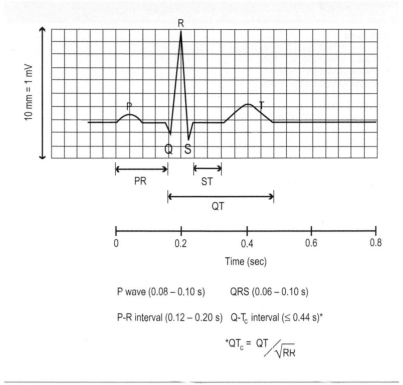

P wave (0.08 – 0.10 s)   QRS (0.06 – 0.10 s)

P-R interval (0.12 – 0.20 s)   Q-T$_c$ interval ($\leq$ 0.44 s)*

$$*QT_c = QT \Big/ \sqrt{RR}$$

Fig. 3.5 ECG trace with grid to allow analysis.

Table 3.4 Alternative method for calculating cardiac axis using leads I–III

ECG lead	Normal	Right axis deviation (RAD)	Left axis deviation (LAD)
Lead I	Positive	Negative	Positive
Lead II	Positive	Positive/negative	Negative
Lead III	Positive/negative	Positive	Negative

- Left axis deviation (aVF predominantly negative) – consider left ventricular hypertrophy (LVH), myocardial infarction (MI).
- Right axis deviation (lead I predominantly negative) – consider coronary heart disease (CHD), right ventricular hypertrophy (RVH).
- The ECG must always be analyzed in its clinical context.

Left ventricular hypertrophy (Box 3.1)
Consider aortic stenosis, hypertension, hypertrophic cardiomyopathy.

Box 3.1 **Criteria for left ventricular hypertrophy on ECG**

Limb leads
- R wave in lead I plus S wave in lead III >25 mm
- R wave in lead aVL >11 mm
- R wave in lead aVF >20 mm
- S wave in lead aVR >14 mm

Precordial leads
- R wave in leads V4, V5 or V6 >26 mm
- R wave in leads V5 or V6 plus S wave in lead V1 >35 mm
- Largest R wave plus largest S wave in precordial leads >45 mm

---

Myocardial ischaemia
ST–elevation myocardial infarct (STEMI)
Defined by chest pain with ECG features as listed in Box 3.2 (see Fig. 3.6). In STEMI, ST elevation morphology evolves over time. Initially there are hyperacute ST changes, followed by the development of Q waves and T wave changes over days (Fig. 3.7).

Non-STEMI
May result in ST segment depression (Fig. 3.8), transient ST elevation or T wave inversion. T wave changes are sensitive for ischaemia but less specific. T waves may become tall, flattened, inverted or biphasic.

Box 3.2 **ECG criteria for ST elevation myocardial infarction**

- Persistent ST segment elevation of ≥1 mm in two contiguous limb leads
- ST segment elevation of ≥2 mm in two contiguous chest leads
- New left bundle branch block

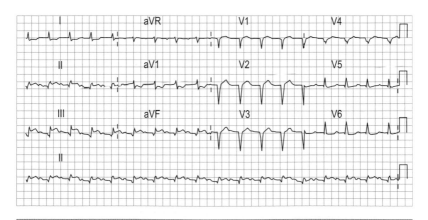

Fig. 3.6 An ECG showing STEMI in the anterior chest leads.

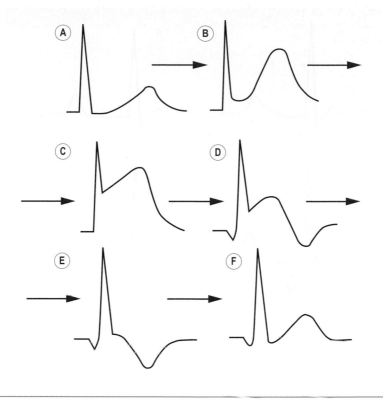

Fig. 3.7 Evolution of acute MI.

Inverted T waves are normal in leads III, aVR and V1, in association with a predominantly negative QRS complex. T waves that are deep and symmetrically inverted strongly suggest myocardial ischaemia.

Q waves (Fig. 3.9) are pathological/abnormal if:
- >1/3 amplitude R wave (in mm)
- >1 mm (40 milliseconds) in duration and/or
- present in the right precordial leads (V1–3).

They represent old MI/scar if in contiguous lead territories (see below).

Correlation between ECG leads and infarct territory
- Leads II, III and aVF – inferior (right coronary artery (RCA) or circumflex artery if nondominant RCA).
- Leads V1 to V3 – anteroseptal (left anterior descending artery).
- Leads I, aVL, V4–V6 – anterolateral (circumflex or dominant RCA).

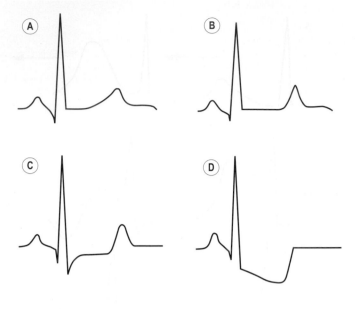

Fig. 3.8 The various forms of ST depression: normal (A), flattened (B), planar (C) and downsloping (D).

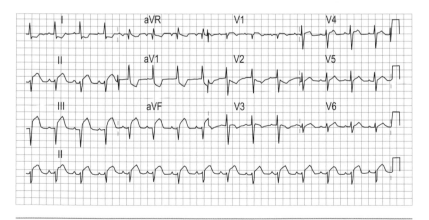

Fig. 3.9 ECG showing inferior lead ST elevation (i, iii, AVF) and the development of Q-waves.

Test: Exercise tolerance test (ETT)

Indications

- Noninvasive investigation for coronary ischaemia – sensitivity of ETT for detecting multivessel disease ~81%. Most useful in patients with an intermediate likelihood of disease based on age, gender and symptoms.
- Risk stratification in patients post MI – as a predictor of the likelihood of a future cardiac event. Patients who achieve an estimated 7 METs (metabolic equivalent) or a heart rate of >130 beats/min in the absence of ischaemic ECG changes (ST depression) are considered low risk.
- Risk stratification of patients with hypertrophic cardiomyopathy – its negative predictive value for sudden death is 97% and in the young, in the absence of other risk factors, permits accurate reassurance.

Contraindications

Acute myocardial ischaemia, severe congestive cardiac failure, severe aortic stenosis, sustained ventricular arrhythmias, severe hypertension (systolic pressure >200, diastolic >110).

How it is done

Exercise on a treadmill/bicycle with simultaneous recording of heart rate, blood pressure and ECG. The Bruce protocol has seven 3-minute stages with increasing speed and incline. It aims to achieve a heart rate response of 85% predicted (220 − age).

The Modified Bruce protocol starts at a lower workload than the standard test, and is typically used for elderly or sedentary patients. The first two stages of the Modified Bruce Test are performed at a 1.7 mph and 0% grade and 1.7 mph and 5% grade, and the third stage corresponds to the first stage of the Standard Bruce Test protocol.

Data presented as

- Symptoms.
- Basic ECG interpretation.
- Reported reason for stopping test.
- Estimate of exercise capacity in METs.
- Blood pressure response.
- Presence of arrhythmias.
- ST changes (type and location).

Interpretation

Exercise test interpretation (Table 3.5)

Limitations

Diagnostic accuracy of the ETT is reduced by any abnormality in the resting 12-lead ECG – left ventricular hypertrophy, right ventricular hypertrophy, bundle branch block and pre-existing ST/T changes.

Meta-analysis of the exercise test studies with angiographic correlates have demonstrated the standard ST response (1 mm depression) to have an average sensitivity of 68% and a specificity of 72% and a predictive accuracy of 69%.

Test: Biochemical markers of myocardial ischaemia

See Fig. 3.10.

Table 3.5 **Exercise test interpretation**	
Results	**Interpretation**
• Target heart rate achieved (220 − age men, 200 − age women) • Normal blood pressure response (increases) • No chest pain • No ST changes	Normal or negative
• Hypotension (>10 mmHg drop in BP in stage 1 or 2) • ≥1 mm downsloping ST depression • >1 mm ST elevation • >2 mm upsloping ST depression • U wave inversion	A positive test

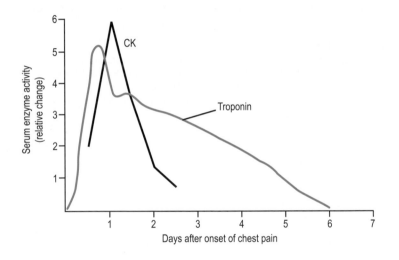

Fig. 3.10 Time course of cardiac enzyme elevations.

Test: Troponin (normal range: Trop T 0.04–0.06 ng/mL, Trop I <0.01 ng/mL)

A complex made of three distinct proteins (I, T and C). In health the cardiac troponins are not detectable. They are highly sensitive markers of myocyte necrosis and are now in common usage. A blood sample is taken for monoclonal antibody testing to cardiac-specific troponin I and cardiac-specific troponin T 12 hours after onset of chest pain, and is currently the most widely used biochemical marker of myocardial injury.

Indications

To aid diagnosis of myocardial infarction. The troponin assay has prognostic information that can determine mortality risk in acute coronary syndromes (ACS) and guides urgency of angiographic intervention.

Limitations

False Positives – troponin and CK may be raised after prolonged arrhythmia, myocarditis, significant LVF and in patients with renal failure and pulmonary embolism.

Test: Creatinine-kinase-MB(CKMB) (Normal range 32–190 IU/L)

Until recently CKMB was the most commonly used iso-enzyme to detect myocardial injury. It remains a useful measure to determine re-infarction, as levels fall to normal only after 36–72 hours.

Echocardiography

Test: Transthoracic echocardiography (TTE) and transoesophageal echocardiography (TOE)

Indications

Structural and functional assessment of the heart and great vessels (Table 3.6).

Table 3.6 **Echo parameters and clinical significance**	
Normal values	**Comment**
Left atrial diameter 3–4 cm	Atrial dilatation can be due to atrioventricular valvular pathology, diastolic dysfunction, interatrial shunts (consider if ventricular function is normal)
Left ventricular (LV) internal diameter (cm): diastole 3.5–5.9, systole 2.4–4.0	LV diastolic dimensions are increased if there is volume loading e.g AR, MR or cardiomyopathy.
LV thickness (cm): septum 0.0–1.3 males, 0.7–1.0 females	Septal thickening is seen in hypertrophic cardiomyopathy (usually 4–6 mm thicker)
LV ejection fraction ≥65%	50–65% mild impairment, 40–50% moderate impairment, <35% severe impairment
Fractional shortening 28–44%	Another quantitative assessment of contractility.

How it is done

- TOE – NBM, sedated, patient supine flat.
- TTE – awake/asleep, semirecumbent.

Physical principles

High-frequency vibration (1–10 MHz) emitted and received from a probe containing a series of piezo-electric crystals. Wave reflection occurs at interfaces between tissues of varying acoustic density and as the speed of ultrasound waves is known, the depth to the reflected surface can be calculated, when the time delay between emission and reception is known. This is displayed as a point on a screen, the magnitude of the point reflecting the strength of reflected signal and is known as B-mode scanning.

There are several imaging modalities but 2D and Doppler have the greatest utility in clinical medicine:

- **2D scanning** (Fig. 3.11) refers to real-time imaging in two-dimensional views with multiple B-mode lines.

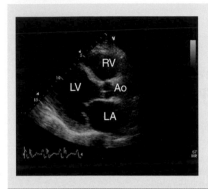

Fig. 3.11 Parasternal long axis view.

- **Doppler scanning** (Fig. 3.12) utilizes the change in frequency observed when ultrasound waves are reflected from a moving target (red blood cells). Change in wavelength is proportional to velocity. Blood flow can be measured at a precise distance from the ultrasound probe with pulsed wave Doppler (PWD), or at all points along the ultrasound beam, without localization known as continuous wave Doppler (CWD).
- **Colour flow Doppler** combines 2D images with PWD to produce a map of blood flow velocities and directions.

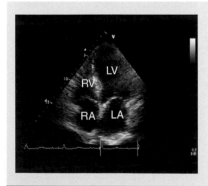

Fig. 3.12 Apical four chamber view.

TTE

Standard views in long axis (LAX) and short axis (SAX) with parasternal, apical, subcostal and occasionally suprasternal positioning. Views can be limited in people with abnormal chest walls or those with a high body mass index.

Assessment of valve function

Aortic stenosis: Assessed by CW Doppler and flow velocity across aortic valve (Table 3.7)

Table 3.7 **Severity of aortic valve disease based on valve pressure gradient**		
Normal	Peak AVG <16 mmHg	nil
Mild	Peak AVG 20–30 mmHg	Mean F AVG <20 mmHg
Moderate	Peak AVG 31–50 mmHg	Mean AVG 20–30 mmHg
Severe	Peak AVG >70 mmHg	Mean AVG 40 mmHg

AVG, aortic valve gradient.

Valve gradient estimated by calculation – $4(V^2)$. The gradient is accurate if LV function is normal. In the presence of impaired LV function the gradient will be underestimated.

Mitral stenosis (Table 3.8)

Based on calculation of mitral valve gradient (MVG mmHg) or mitral valve area (MVA cm^2).

Table 3.8 **Severity of mitral valve disease based on valve pressure gradient**	
Mild	Mean MVG <5 mmHg
Moderate	Mean MVG 5–10 mmHg
Severe	Mean MVG >10 mmHg

MVG, mitral valve gradient.

Mitral regurgitation (Table 3.9)

Based on analysis of colour flow Doppler (CFD) and Continuous wave Doppler (CWD) profile. Graded from 1 (mild) to 4 (severe). Please see Table 3.9.

Table 3.9 **Grading of regurgitation for mitral and aortic valve**		
0/4	None	No regurgitation
1/4	Mild	Regurgitant flow limited to immediately around the valve area
2/4	Moderate	Regurgitant flow occupies up to a third of the chamber
3/4	Moderate to severe	Regurgitant flow occupies up to 2/3 of the chamber
4/4	Severe	Regurgitant flow in most of the receiving chamber and flow reversal in pulmonary veins

Aortic regurgitation

Assessed in a similar way to MR, by CFD and CWD (see above):
- the pressure half time of the CWD regurgitant jet is measured and the shorter the half time the more severe the regurgitation
- <240 milliseconds is considered severe.

Limitations (Table 3.10)

Echocardiography is operator dependent and with TOE there is a 1–2% risk of significant complication including respiratory compromise, emesis, agitation, oesophageal rupture, haemorrhage and cardiac dysrhythmia.

Interobserver variation and false-positive tests may be common if the clinical question is not focused.

Table 3.10 **Comparison of TTE and TOE**		
Clinical indication	TTE useful	TOE useful
Atria and ventricle size, shape and function	+	+
Pericardial effusion	−	+
Myocardial thickness	+	+
Valve structure and function	+	++
Aortic arch	+	Limited
Left atrial appendage	−	+
Superior vena cava	Limited	+
Thoracic aorta	−	+
Clinical utility		
Noninvasive	+	−
Image quality operator dependent	+	−
Can be performed in sitting position	+	−
Sedation required	−	+

Cardiac catheterization

Test: Coronary angiography

Indication
- Diagnostic: the assessment of the coronary circulation.
- Therapeutic: percutaneous coronary intervention (PCI) with angioplasty (PTCA) or stenting in the acute or elective setting.

How it is done
X-ray guided with arterial access via the radial, brachial or femoral artery. Catheter manipulated in coronary arteries or coronary graft ostia. Iodinated contrast and radiological imaging capture standard views.

Data presented as

Images capture flow of contrast in coronary circulation and significant atheromatous narrowings in the arteries may be seen (Fig. 3.13).

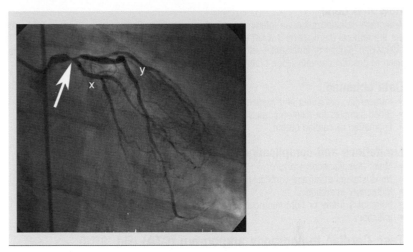

Fig. 3.13 Left mainstem stenosis (arrow) on coronary angiogram. y, left anterior descending (LAD); x, circumflex artery.

Interpretation

Flow-limiting stenoses >60% are considered significant, but should be interpreted in a clinical context.

Management principles

1. Discrete lesions, which correlate with proven ischaemic territories (on ECG, echo or stress testing), may be amenable to angioplasty and stenting.
2. Multiple stenoses (particularly if the left main-stem) should be considered for surgery.
3. Diffuse disease not suitable for intervention is managed with medical therapy alone.

Limitations and complications

- Risk of serious complication ≤1/1000 (more for acute coronary revascularization).
- Bleeding and haematoma formation at the cannulation site.
- Cerebrovascular events (plaque embolization).
- Dissection of the coronary artery.
- Cardiac arrhythmia.
- Contrast agent nephropathy.

Test: Right heart catheterization

Indications

- Measurement and analysis of right heart, pulmonary artery and pulmonary capillary wedge pressures.
- Measurement of cardiac output by thermodilution.
- Screening for intracardiac shunts.

- Temporary ventricular pacing.
- Assessment of arrhythmias.
- Pulmonary wedge angiography.

How it is done

Antegrade catheterization via inferior or superior vena cava. Percutaneous entry is achieved via the femoral (particularly if a left heart catheter is being done at the same time), subclavian, jugular or antecubital vein. Balloon flotation catheters or fluoroscopic guidance is used to position catheters (see Chapter 9).

Data obtained

- Intracardiac pressures and oxygen saturations.
- Blood samples for oximetric analysis and shunts diagnosis.
- Estimation of cardiac output.

Limitations and complications

- Major complications are rare.
- Nonsustained atrial and ventricular arrhythmias are common.
- Pulmonary infarction.
- Pulmonary artery or right ventricular perforation.
- Infection.

Test: Cardiac tomography angiogram (CTA) (Fig. 3.14)

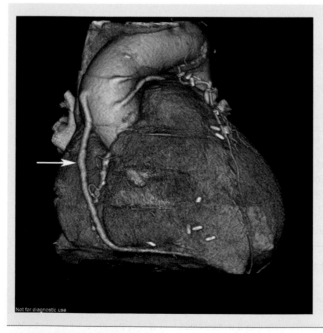

Not for diagnostic use

Fig. 3.14 CT angiogram showing saphenous vein graft (arrow).

Indications
- For diagnostic work-up of patients with typical angina pectoris.
- To detect and exclude significant coronary disease with high negative predictive value.
- May obviate the need for invasive coronary angiography.

How it is done
Noninvasive contrast CT. Scan takes approximately 30 seconds to perform.

Data presented as
2D image.

Interpretation
A 'normal' CT coronary angiogram allows the clinician to rule out the presence of haemodynamically relevant coronary artery stenoses with a high degree of reliability.

Limitations
Patients often require drugs to slow the heart for image acquisition. This is a relatively new diagnostic tool. CTA has a sensitivity of 89%, a specificity of 65%, a positive predictive value (PPV) of 13% and a negative predictive value (NPV) of 99% for detecting >50% stenosis, compared with gold-standard angiography.

Further investigations
Hybrid positron emission tomography CT (PET-CT) and single photon emission computed tomography (SPECT-CT) allow for the acquisition of metabolic and/or perfusion information as well as anatomic data, and has promise as a future diagnostic tool.

Nuclear imaging

Test: Thallium/technetium scan (Fig. 3.15)

Indication
Diagnostic
- Assessment of coronary artery disease in those with inability to exercise or where an abnormal resting ECG makes interpretation of ST changes difficult, e.g. left bundle branch block (LBBB).
- Assessment of patients with recurrence of symptoms post revascularization.

Prognostic
- Risk stratification in patients before noncardiac surgery.
- Noninvasive testing for inducible ischaemia.
- Assessment of myocardial viability prior to revascularization.

How it is done
- Radiolabelled tracers (e.g. thallium-201) is injected peripherally and is taken up by myocytes.
- Radioactivity detected by gamma camera.
- Tracer distribution proportional to blood flow.

Interpretation
Areas of ischaemia or infarction take up less thallium. Between 2 and 24 hours post injection, cardiac myocytes contain a comparable concentration (the thallium redistributes in areas with viable myocardium). Images at this time show dark areas where the myocardium has infarcted, but normal density in ischaemic areas. By comparing the early and late images

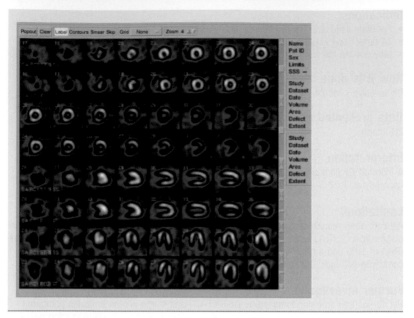

Fig. 3.15 A thallium scan.

one can predict whether an ischaemic area of myocardium contains enough viable tissue to warrant intervention.

Test: Technetium-99-labelled sestamibi

Technetium-99-labelled sestamibi (MIBI) does not undergo redistribution. When injected during exercise, its distribution in the myocardium indicates the distribution of blood during exercise, even if the image is taken several hours later. The images produced following injection of Tc 99m during exercise can be compared to images produced following injection at rest in order to determine which areas of ischaemia are reversible. In patients unable to exercise, the heart rate can be increased by pharmacological agents, e.g. dipyridamole or dobutamine.

Technetium tracers are higher energy and are less affected by attenuation. These tracers can also be used for acquiring multiple images of the cardiac cycle (cardiac gating), which enables ejection fraction to be estimated. They also identify wall motion abnormalities.

Limitations

Thallium is a low-energy tracer – this can result in soft tissue attenuation (e.g. by overlying breast tissue) which can produce a false-positive scan. Stress perfusion scans are positive in 75% to 90% of patients with anatomically significant coronary disease and in 20% to 30% of those without it.

Test: Cardiac MRI (CMR) (Fig. 3.16)

Indications

- Congenital heart disease.
- Cardiomyopathy/infiltrative myocardial disease (e.g. sarcoid)/pericarditis.

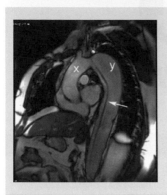

Fig. 3.16 A cardiac MRI showing an aortic dissection. x, ascending aorta; y, descending aorta; arrow, dissection flap).

- Disease of the aorta.
- Valvular heart disease.
- Coronary artery disease.
- Pulmonary vessel imaging.

How it is done

CMR scanners employ cardiac and respiratory gating to effectively suspend cardiorespiratory motion. It provides still or moving images that are both anatomical and functional.

Intravenous gadolinium can be used with a myocardial perfusion study, contrast enhanced angiography or for myocardial infarct imaging.

Limitations and complications

Contraindications are metallic implants or debris, permanent pacemakers or defibrillators, intracerebral clips and significant claustrophobia.

TOPIC ④

Central nervous system

Topic Contents

Assessment of consciousness 58
Test: Glasgow Coma Scale (GCS) 58
CSF analysis 60
Test: Lumbar puncture 60
Test: CSF appearance
(spectrophotometry) 61
Test: CSF cell counts 62
Test: CSF glucose 63
Test: CSF microbiology 64
Test: CSF opening pressure 64
Test: CSF protein 64
Electroencephalogram
derivatives 65
Test: Bispectral index (BIS) 66

Evoked potentials 68
Test: Somatosensory evoked potentials
(SSEPs) 69
Test: Motor evoked potentials (MEPs) 70
Test: Auditory evoked potentials (AEPs) 71
Imaging 73
Test: Computerized tomography (CT) brain 73
Test: MRI brain 75
Cervical spine in trauma 77
Test: Plain cervical radiographs 77
Test: Cervical CT scan 80
Test: Cervical MRI 81
Intracranial pressure (ICP) monitoring 81
Malignant hyperthermia susceptibility 85

Assessment of consciousness

Test: Glasgow Coma Scale (GCS)

Indications
- Assessment of consciousness initially used after traumatic brain injury but now also applied to other situations.

How it is done
- Sum the scores of the three eye, verbal and motor tests (Tables 4.1 and 4.2).

Interpretation
Data presented as a final score.
- The highest score is 15 with a fully awake patient.
- The lowest possible score is 3 when patients are dead or in deep coma.
- Ideally the breakdown of the separate components should be recorded.

  Causes of reduced GCS include:
- Acute brain injury: traumatic, vascular and infections
- Metabolic disorders: hypoglycaemia, hepatic or renal failure
- Drugs: including sedatives and alcohol.

Table 4.1 Glasgow coma scale scores for the three tests, plus variables in children

Best eye response

Score	Description
4	Eyes open spontaneously
3	Eyes open to speech. Do not confuse with arousal of sleeping patient
2	Eyes open to pain. Try fingernail bed pressure. Supraorbital pressure will cause grimace and eye closure
1	No eye opening, ensure painful stimulus is adequate

Best verbal response

Score	Description
5	Orientated in time, person and place
4	Responds to questions but is disorientated and confused
3	Inappropriate, random words
2	Incomprehensible sounds and moans but no words
1	None

Verbal response is adjusted in children

Score	Verbal response	Preverbal/grimace response
5	Appropriate babbles, words or phrases to usual ability	Normal facial oromotor activity
4	Inappropriate words, or spontaneous irritable cry	Less than usual ability, response only to touch
3	Cries inappropriately	Vigorous grimace to pain
2	Grunts to pain, occasional whimpers	Mild grimace to pain
1	No vocal response	No response to pain

Best motor response, test and record in each limb*

Score	Description
6	Obeys commands
5	Localizes pain. Hand should cross midline or get above clavicle in attempt to remove the stimulus
4	Withdraws from pain. Pulls limb away from fingernail bed pressure. Normal flexion observed
3	Abnormal flexion, decorticate response (spastic wrist flexion)
2	Extension to pain, decerebrate response (extensor posturing)
1	No motor response. Ensure adequate painful stimulus and no spinal injury

*Upper limb responses are more reliable as lower limb responses could be spinal reflexes.

Table 4.2 **Severity of acute head injury**	
GCS score	Coma
≤ 8	Severe
9–12	Moderate
≤ 13	Minor

Management principles
- Patients with a GCS of 8 or less should be intubated to ensure airway protection, oxygenation and CO_2 clearance.
- NICE guidelines advise the frequency of the observations after traumatic brain injury.

Limitations and complications
- Failure to incorporate brainstem reflexes.
- It is most accurate in assessing altered levels of consciousness due to trauma, but is often used to assess medical causes of coma.
- The presence of an endotracheal tube precludes use of the verbal assessment. 'T' is then recorded in this section (e.g. $M_5 \, V_T \, E_3$).
- In spinal cord injury the stimulation and assessment of the motor response needs to be applied above the level of injury.
- Orbital trauma may prevent assessment of eye opening.

CSF analysis

Test: Lumbar puncture

Indications
- Diagnostic Lumbar Puncture.

Analysis of CSF is required for the diagnosis of the following CNS conditions:
- Infections, including bacterial, viral and fungal meningitis, Inflammatory CNS disease; including encephalitis, myelitis, Guillain Barré syndrome and multiple sclerosis, CNS malignancy, and Intracerebral haemorrhage.
- Reduce CSF volume for therapeutic purposes.
- Administer intrathecal drugs, e.g. chemotherapy, spinal anaesthesia, etc.,

Conditions in which lumbar punctures are commonly undertaken include:
- Infection, including bacterial, viral and fungal meningitis
- Inflammatory CNS disease; including encephalitis, myelitis, Guillain Barré syndrome and multiple sclerosis.
- CNS malignancy.
- Intracerebral haemorrhage.

Contraindications
- Reduced GCS.
- Focal neurological signs.
- Papilloedema.
- Coagulation disorders.
- Local infection at site.

Normal values
See Table 4.3

Table 4.3 **Lumbar puncture results**	
Measure	Normal values
Opening pressure	7–20 cmH$_2$0
Cell count	0–5/mm^3, all lymphocytes
Protein concentration	0.15–0.45 g/L
Glucose concentration	2.8–4.2 mmol/L
CSF: blood glucose ratio	65%

Limitations and complications
- Headache:
    - Incidence of post dural puncture headache (PDPH) is reduced with smaller needle size. The average frequency of headache is 20–40% using 20–22 G and 5–12% using 24–27 G needles
    - Incidence also reduced by using a noncutting (Whittacre or Sprotte) type needle rather than cutting (Quinke) type, and by replacement of stylet before needle withdrawal. There is no evidence increased fluids or bed rest prevents headache.
- Traumatic tap – defined as CSF containing >1000 RBC per high-powered field.
- Backache – may occur in up to 40% of patients.
- Failure.
- Spinal cord or nerve root damage–replacement of stylet before needle withdrawal may avoid damage to nerve roots and dura.
- Cerebral herniation is rare and can be avoided by using CT to exclude a space-occupying lesion (SOL) prior to lumbar puncture.
- Subdural, epidural haematomas.
- Cranial nerve palsies.
- Discitis.
- Pneumocephalus.
- Infection.

Test: CSF appearance (spectrophotometry)
- Xanthrochromia is the yellowish discoloration of Cerebrospinal fluid (CSF) due to the presence of bilirubin, a haemoglobin breakdown product.
- Visual inspection alone is not a reliable method to detect xanthochromia. Spectrophotometry is necessary.

Indications
- In a suspected subarachnoid haemorrhage (SAH), an LP should be done ideally 12 hours after the suspected haemorrhage to allow for the in vivo formation of CSF bilirubin.

How it is done
- If possible collect four sequential CSF specimens and ensure the last sample is sent for bilirubin analysis.

- Check with the laboratory for the volume required and ensure availability of spectrophotometry.
- Protect sample from light and when possible avoid vacuum transport systems that may haemolyze red blood cells (RBCs), produce oxyhaemoglobin (oxyHb) and hence a false-positive result.
- A simultaneous blood specimen should be taken for serum bilirubin and total protein.
- After centrifugation the supernatant is analyzed with a spectrophotometer.
- Haem pigments produce characteristic absorbance peaks at 400–460 nm.

Interpretation
Normal CSF appearance is crystal clear and colourless

Abnormalities
- Need to be interpreted carefully as causes of xanthochromia include raised serum bilirubin and CSF protein.
- The exact ratios of RBC, oxyHb and bilirubin found in the CSF will depend upon the timing of the lumbar puncture in relationship to the bleed.
- If a CT scan and CSF spectrophotometry are normal within 2 weeks of a sudden severe headache then SAH is excluded.

Further investigations
- Patients with a CT positive for subarachnoid blood should proceed to either a cerebral angiogram or CT angiogram to try and find the cause of the SAH (an aneurysm in >85% of cases). Treatment can then be undertaken (surgical or radiological) with the aim of preventing a re-bleed and allowing the aggressive management of vasospasm.
- The small group of patients with a history suggestive of a SAH but with a negative CT, can be identified with an appropriately timed lumbar puncture followed by spectrophotometer CSF analysis. They can then also be referred for cerebral angiography.

Limitations and complications
- Sensitivity of bilirubin to diagnose a subarachnoid haemorrhage has been shown to be 96% when undertaken more than 12 hours after haemorrhage.
- A traumatic tap will produce a CSF sample with an increased RBC count, but unlike SAH the sample will not contain bilirubin. Spectrophotometry is the only reliable way to distinguish SAH from a traumatic tap.
- Spectrophotometric findings taken on a second or subsequent LP only reflect the probability that blood has been introduced into the subarachnoid space at an earlier puncture.

Test: CSF cell counts
Indications
- Diagnostic lumbar puncture.
- Monitoring of partially treated meningitis/ventriculitis.

How it is done
- Cell count must be performed manually by an experienced operator using a Neubauer chamber within 30 minutes of sampling.
- White blood cell (WBC) differential is usually performed on concentrated CSF by centrifugation.

Interpretation
Normal range
- Adults <5 WBC/mm^3 (70% lymphocytes, 30% monocytes, occasional eosinophil or neutrophil).
- Neonates <20 WBC/mm^3, including <60% neutrophils.

Abnormalities
See Table 4.4.

Table 4.4 Causes of elevated CSF white blood cell count	
	Characteristics
Bacterial meningitis	Often >1000/mm^3, usually PMN
Viral meningitis	<100/mm^3, usually lymphocytes
Seizures	
Intracerebral haemorrhage	
Malignancy	
Guillain-Barré syndrome	<50 monocytes/mm^3
Multiple sclerosis	<50 monocytes/mm^3
Other inflammatory conditions	

WBC differential

Viral, fungal and tuberculosis (TB) infections characteristically show lymphocytosis, but early infection may show polymorphonuclear neutrophil (PMN) preponderance. Eosinophilic meningitis >10 eosinophils/mm^3 is rare. Causes include parasitic infections, other infections, VP shunts, malignancy and allergic drug reactions.

Limitations and complications

- Cell counts diminish after 30 minutes due to settling, binding to surfaces and cell lysis. Neutrophil counts fall by 50% by 2 hours whereas lymphocytes and monocytes do not.
- Allow 1 WBC per 500 RBCs in the event of traumatic tap.

Test: CSF glucose (Table 4.5)

Table 4.5 Causes of altered CSF glucose	
Low CSF glucose	High CSF glucose
CNS infections	Hyperglycaemia
Chemical meningitis	
Subarachnoid haemorrhage	
Hypoglycaemia	

Interpretation

Normal range
- CSF glucose should be approximately two-thirds serum glucose: a simultaneous serum sample should always be taken.
- Levels rarely go above 17 mmol/L regardless of serum levels.
- **Beware:** glucose levels are usually normal in viral infections and can be normal in up to 50% of bacterial CNS infections.

Test: CSF microbiology

Indications
- Diagnostic lumbar puncture.

How it is done
- Gram stain for suspected bacterial infections.
- Acid-fast staining for suspected TB.
- India ink stain for cryptococcus.
- CSF culture is essential to determine antimicrobial sensitivity and resistance. A minimum of 2 mL is required. However, fungal and TB cultures require 20–40 mL to provide reasonable sensitivity. This requires multiple CSF samples.
- Polymerase chain reaction (PCR) has replaced tissue culture for most viral and some bacterial CNS disease.
- CSF antigen testing. For cryptococcus this has a sensitivity of 80–95%.
- Latex agglutination and coagglutination are methods that allow detection of bacterial antigens in CSF. For *Haemophilus* influenza sensitivity is quoted to be 60–100%, but is lower for other bacteria. This can be useful in partially treated meningitis where cultures may not yield an organism.

Test: CSF opening pressure

Indications
- All lumbar punctures.

How it is done
- Connect manometer to lumbar puncture needle hub once CSF is draining. Allow CSF pressure to equilibrate with atmospheric pressure in the manometer tubing.
- Read the pressure in cmH_2O/mmH_2O calibrated onto manometer tubing.

Interpretation
Normal data (Table 4.6)

Table 4.6 **Normal range of CSF pressure**	
Age (years)	Pressure (cmH_2O)
<8	1–10
>8	6–20
Obese adult	<25

Pressures can become elevated if the patient holds their breath or strains. It will reduce with hyperventilation. Fluctuations may be seen with respirations.

Abnormalities
See Table 4.7.

Test: CSF protein

Indications
- CSF protein concentration is one of the most sensitive indicators of pathology within the CNS.

Table 4.7 **Causes of altered CSF pressure**	
High pressure ($>$25 cmH$_2$O)	Low pressure ($<$6 cmH$_2$O)
Intracranial haemorrhage	CSF leak
Space-occupying lesions	Previous lumbar puncture
Meningitis	Severe dehydration
Cerebral oedema	Inadequate production
Congestive cardiac failure	Shunt
High venous pressure	Obstructive hydrocephalus Excess absorption
Idiopathic/benign intracranial hypertension	Drugs: acetazolamide, diuretics

Interpretation

Normal range
- Adult range 0.15–0.45 g/L is reached between 6 and 12 months of age.
- Newborns have up to 1.5 g/L.

Abnormalities (Table 4.8)
- CSF: serum ratio of albumin is 1:200. Immunoglobulins are normally excluded from CSF; their CSF:serum ratio is $>$1:500 and essentially consists only of IgG.
- Oligoclonal bands present in the CSF but not serum suggest an immune response within CNS.
- CSF protein levels $>$2 g/L suggest bacterial infections.

Table 4.8 **Causes of altered CSF protein**	
Elevated CSF protein	Low CSF protein
Infections	Repeated LP
Intracranial haemorrhage	Chronic CSF leak
Multiple sclerosis	Children 6 months to 2 years
Guillain-Barré syndrome	Acute water intoxication
Malignancy	
Endocrine abnormalities	
Drugs	

Limitations and complications
- Allow 0.01 g/L protein for every 1000 RBCs/mm^3 in the event of a traumatic tap.
- Measurement is technique dependent; check own laboratory reference range.

Electroencephalogram derivatives

The electroencephalogram (EEG) is produced from the electrical activity in the superficial cerebral cortex. Scalp electrodes are used, the exact location of which has been determined by an international system. Each electrode can detect activity within 2.5 cm. The resulting signal is amplified, filtered and then displayed visually on a plot of amplitude versus time. Computerized Fourier analysis can be undertaken to show amplitude at each frequency, power versus frequency or a compressed spectral array.

Monitors that use the EEG include the bispectral index, cerebral state index, patient state index, narcotrend index and spectral entropy monitors.

Test: Bispectral index (BIS)

Indications

- To attempt to reduce the incidence of awareness during anaesthesia.
- Monitoring hypnosis/depth of anaesthesia.
- Titrate sedation/anaesthesia to reduce side effects.

How it is done

- A single adhesive probe with four sensors is attached over the frontal cortex.
- The probe is connected to the BIS software and a single figure is displayed on screen.
- The BIS is a dimensionless number ranging from 100 (fully awake) to 0 (isoelectric EEG, deep coma). It is calculated from bispectral EEG analysis.
- The BIS calculates subparameters including beta ratio, SynchFastSlow and burst suppression.
  - *Beta ratio* is the log ratio of the power in high and medium frequency bands: this is most influential during light hypnotic states with characteristic high β activity.
  - *SynchFastSlow* is the relative bispectral power in the 40–47 Hz frequency band: this predominates during surgical levels of anaesthesia.
  - *Burst suppression ratio (SR)* is the proportion of isoelectric 'suppressed' EEG in the preceding 1 minute. Increasing anaesthetic drug concentrations gives increasing duration of suppressed periods with intermittent high frequency high amplitude 'burst' activity. This detects very deep anaesthesia.
- The analysis uses an algorithm that produces a linear relationship between the numerical BIS value and the concentration of sedative.

Interpretation

Abnormalities
- It is advisable to confirm a normal BIS value in patients before induction of anaesthesia, although this is often not undertaken.
- Low voltage EEG occurs occasionally, which can be misinterpreted as burst suppression.

Physiological principles
See Fig. 4.1.

Management principles

- There is currently no gold standard measure of anaesthetic depth.
- Practioners administer anaesthetic agents to keep the BIS value between 40 and 60, generally considered to indicate adequate depth of anaesthesia.
- BIS is drug dependent and no specific BIS value can *guarantee* unconsciousness, but there is evidence that its use is associated with a reduction in awareness under anaesthesia.

Limitations and complications

Drugs
- Nitrous oxide (N_2O) generally does not alter BIS values, but case reports have shown variable effects.

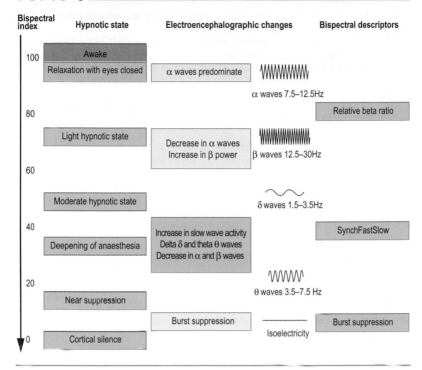

Fig. 4.1 Physiological principles of bispectral index measurement. (Reproduced with permission from Dahaba AA (2005) Anaesth Analg 101:765-773.)

- Ketamine causes an increase in the β activity accompanied by a reduction in the δ power. This different EEG pattern is reflected by a BIS increase after ketamine administration.
- Opioids at analgesic concentrations do not produce BIS/EEG alterations on the cerebral cortex.
- Suxamethonium causes artefact decrease of BIS values.
- Aminophylline and doxapram will increase BIS values and speed recovery.
- Different anaesthetic drugs have different EEG changes. BIS values may not be the same when using different combinations of anaesthetic agents.

Interference

The following produce interference and have been reported to increase BIS values: electrocautery, pacemakers, forced air warming blankets, endoscopic shaver oscillators, electromagnetic positioning systems and ECG. Newer monitors may be less susceptible to electrical interference.

Clinical conditions

- Hypothermia produces slowing of the EEG below 35°C. Electrical silence occurs between 7 and 20°C.
- Hypoglycaemia can produce a pattern similar to general anaesthesia with BIS values as low as 45. BIS values will increase as blood glucose is restored and consciousness is returned.

- Cerebral ischaemia will cause EEG slowing. Cortical silence can occur within 20 seconds given complete absence of cerebral blood flow.
- A BIS value of 0 has been shown to accurately indicate brain death in the presence of other confirmatory tests of brainstem death.
- Further clinical causes of abnormal EEG patterns include post ictus, Alzheimer's dementia, cerebral palsy and severe brain injury. Their exact effect upon BIS values has not yet been quantified.
- Performance of BIS has not been studied extensively in the presence of concomitant medications including antidepressants, anticonvulsants and analgesics.

Other limitations

- There are differences in the EEG of children compared to adults. As a result BIS values in children show a much wider spread, and it is unclear if this index can be used to determine depth of anaesthesia in children.
- The algorithm used varies with different models of monitor. This may improve resistance to artefacts but give different BIS values depending on the model used.
- BIS values do not predict the likelihood of movement.
- Case reports have been published of explicit recall despite adequate BIS readings.

Evoked potentials

Evoked potentials (EP) measure action potentials that occur in response to a specific stimulus. The recorded potentials test a specific neural tract, sensory or motor, peripheral or central. Evoked potentials are smaller than EEG and require computer averaging to resolve them from background signals (EEG and ECG). The EP waveform (Fig. 4.2) is a plot of voltage versus time. It is described in terms of amplitude, latency and morphology.

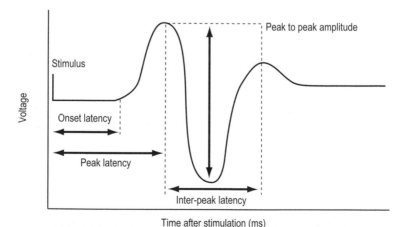

Fig. 4.2 Schematic diagram of an evoked potential.

Guidelines and standards are available from The International Federation of Clinical Neurophysiology at http://www.ifcn.info/ and The American Clinical Neurophysiology Society at http://www.acns.org/.

Intraoperative monitoring should be considered whenever the function of the brain, brainstem, spinal cord or selected peripheral nerve is at risk. This includes surgery for scoliosis, spinal trauma, spinal cord pathologies, tethered cords, brainstem tumours, cranial nerve involvement and thoracoabdominal aortic aneurysms.

Test: Somatosensory evoked potentials (SSEPs)

Indications

- To assess central sensory function and the integrity of the sensory tract.
- To possibly reduce neurological deficit post scoliosis surgery.
- Diagnostic spinal cord injury studies.
- During carotid endarterectomy (CEA) for cortical protection and thus an indication for shunt placement.
- During SAH vasospasm, surgical clipping and embolization of spinal cord AVMs.

How it is done

- A peripheral nerve is stimulated using surface electrodes to deliver an electrical stimulus. Nerves usually used are the tibial, common peroneal, median and ulnar nerves. Unilateral stimulation is usually used with stimuli alternated between legs.
- The stimulus intensity is adjusted to produce a consistent muscle twitch or maximal cortical SEP amplitude.
- The EP is recorded at various points along the neural pathway using surface or needle electrodes.
- Spinal potentials are recorded over cervical and lumbar spinous processes. They may be recorded invasively using epidural or surgically placed wire electrodes.
- Subcortical potentials are recorded over C2 vertebrae.
- Cortical SSEPs are recorded from standard scalp EEG electrodes.

Interpretation

Data presented as

- Generally amplitude reduction of >50% or latency increase of 10% is usually considered significant.

Physiological principles

- Neuronal activity passes along the nerves, up the ipsilateral dorsal columns, to synapse in the cervicomedullary junction. It crosses the midline, ascends through the contralateral medial lemniscus in the brainstem to synapse again in the thalamus. The final projections reach the parietal sensory cortex.
- Additional components may ascend the spinal cord through the posterior spinocerebellar pathways.

Normal range/graph

See Fig. 4.3.

Abnormalities

- Surgical factors – direct trauma, retraction, compression, stretching, positioning, blood flow impairment and vascular clamps.
- Anaesthetic agents – anaesthetic agents (inhalational and intravenous) and N_2O produce a dose related increased SSEP latency and decreased amplitude.

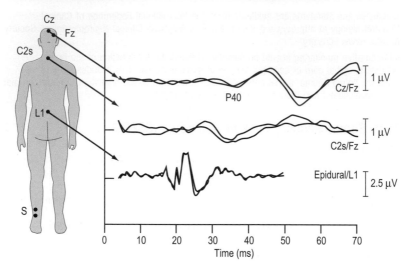

Fig. 4.3 Somatosensory AP normal range/graph.

- Physiological effects – temperature, ischaemia, hypotension, raised ICP, age, and neurological disorders can all result in EP deterioration.
- Equipment and technical problems – good electrical isolation of equipment is essential.

Management principles
- Aim for a stable steady state anaesthetic, using low concentrations of inhalational agents supplemented with opioid infusions (remifentanil) to produce ideal conditions for monitoring.
- Boluses are avoided as interpretation of the following EP is difficult.
- Neuromuscular block may be necessary to prevent compartment syndrome occurring at the site of the SSEP stimulus.

Limitations and complications
- SSEPs may remain intact despite injury to the anterior spinal cord or nerve root injury. To detect this you require EMG or MEP monitoring.
- To reduce false negatives you measure both latency and amplitude, and maximize the number of recording electrodes.
- SSEPs are averaged over 10–40 seconds, which causes delayed warning to the surgical team.

Test: Motor evoked potentials (MEPs)
MEPs assess the motor pathway from the motor cortex to the NMJ. In combination with SSEP monitoring, addition of MEP improves sensitivity and specificity for detecting neuronal injury.

Indications
- When anterior spinal artery blood supply is jeopardized.
- Spinal vascular malformations and spinal cord tumours.

Advantages

- Direct monitoring of motor tract and improved sensitivity for postoperative motor deficits.
- Allows for individual limb assessment.
- No averaging is required thus prompt corrections can be made.

How it is done

- Baseline recordings are made after induction of anaesthesia.
- Stimulation of the motor cortex using electrical or magnetic techniques. (Magnetic stimulation is more difficult in the anaesthetized patient.)
- Transcranial high frequency repetitive stimulus protocols make it possible to elicit MEPs in anaesthetized patients.
- The evoked response is recorded as either a compound muscle action potential (CMAP) in the peripheral muscle or a spinal cord nerve action potential.

Interpretation

Data presented as

- Presence or absence of response, amplitude changes, changes in thresholds or a combination.

Abnormalities

- Preoperative paraplegics will have no recordable MEPs in affected areas.
- MEPs are abolished by neuromuscular blocking drugs, although sometimes partial NMB is requested to reduce background noise.
- MEPs are easily abolished by inhalational anaesthetic agents.

Management principles

- TIVA anaesthetic using propofol and opioids is required as MEPs are abolished by inhalational anaesthetics.
- Cardiovascular stability is crucial as CMAPs are highly sensitive to variation in blood pressure and local blood perfusion.

Limitations and complications

- Tongue/lip bites can occur and require protection with insertion of a bite block.
- Other movement related injuries, burns, arrhythmias and lacerations have been documented. Seizures are rare.
- Epidural electrodes may not monitor motor tracts reliably.

Further investigations

- A wake up test is performed if a change in the recorded evoked potentials occurs and an injury is suspected. This is to check for a clinical deficit.
- EEG may be more useful for detection of cerebral ischaemia.

Test: Auditory evoked potentials (AEPs)

Indications

- Assessment of hearing and VIII cranial nerve function.
- Intraoperative monitoring during cerebellopontine angle surgery, microvascular decompression surgery and posterior fossa tumour removal.
- Monitoring depth of anaesthesia.

How it is done

- Stimulus supplied through headphones – ear receives a clicking sound at intensity 65–70 dB, at repetition 10 Hz.
- Sensor electrodes are placed over the vertex and mastoid process. An extra ground electrode is placed over the forehead.

- The contralateral ear receives noise at 30–40 dB.
- Signal averaging of the EEG yields a sequence of waveforms that corresponds to the neural response along the pathway from the auditory nerve VIII, through the brainstem and to the cortex.

Interpretation
See Fig. 4.4.

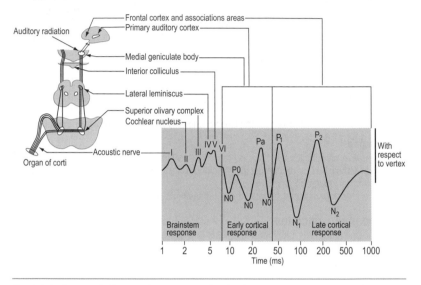

Fig. 4.4 Auditory evoked potential normal range/graph. (Reproduced with permission from Thornton C, Sharpe RM (1998) Evoked responses in anaesthesia 4. Br J Anaesth 81:771–81, and Kumar A, Bhattacharya A, Makhija N (2000) Evoked potential monitoring in anaesthesia and analgesia. Anaesthesia 55:225–41.)

Physiological principles
The waveform allows anatomical location of a dysfunction along the auditory pathway
- Brainstem response (BAEP) <10 ms.
- Early/mid cortical response (MLAEP) 10–80 ms.
- Long latency AEP >80 ms.

Abnormalities
BAEP is used for cochlear, auditory nerve and brainstem function:
- Response is affected by conductive and sensorineural hearing disorders
- Peak latency is affected by age, sex, repetition rate of stimulus, intensity and polarity
- Interpeak latency is increased by hypoglycaemia
- Brainstem death invariably has abnormal brainstem AEPs
- BAEP is generally unaffected by anaesthetics and mild hypothermia.

Mid latency AEP (10–50 ms):
- Inhalational and IV general anaesthetic agents prolong latency and reduce amplitude of waves Pa and Nb in a dose dependent manner
- AEP index is a mathematical derivative of MLAEP waveform. It is a method used to detect the transition from consciousness to unconsciousness.

Further investigations
• Combined use of other evoked potentials or other cranial nerves (facial nerve function) may be required for optimal functional outcome.

Limitations and complications
• The significance of brainstem AEP changes depends upon the surgery.
• Assessment of AEP latencies and amplitudes is done by visual inspection and is subject to observer bias.
• It requires computer averaging, which can take up to 2 minutes. This time lapse limits usefulness during surgical procedures.
• MLAEP is affected by muscle movement, diathermy and electrical interference.
• There is poor agreement among experts regarding signal quality.

Imaging

Test: Computerized tomography (CT) brain
Head injury
NICE guidelines for head injury (http://www.nice.org.uk) were published in 2003 and updated in 2007. The presence of any of the following risk factors requires CT brain imaging following head injury:
• GCS <13 at any point
• GCS 13–14 at 2 hours post injury
• Suspected open or depressed skull fracture
• Any sign of basal skull fracture
• Post-traumatic seizure
• Focal neurological deficit
• >1 episode vomiting
• Amnesia >30 minutes of events before impact
• Additional high-risk patients include those with coagulopathy, age >65 and dangerous mechanism of injury.

For children under two, it is recommended by NICE (2007) that the best evidence currently available is the 'CHALICE' rule (see http://www.nice.org.uk for more details).

How it is done
• CT brain imaging may use a sequential single-slice technique, multislice helical (spiral) protocol or multidetector multislice algorithm.
• Slice thickness <10 mm supratentorial, <5 mm for posterior fossa and children.
• Base of skull slice thickness should be 2–3 mm depending on technique.
• Soft tissue and bony images are required.
• Contrast may be required, e.g. meningioma.

Interpretation
Please see Fig. 4.5 for a normal CT scan.
Abnormalities
• Cerebral oedema: loss of grey-white differentiation, sulcal and ventricular effacement with increased brain volume.
• Subarachnoid haemorrhage (Fig. 4.6): blood in the CSF is seen as hyperdensity in the suprasellar cistern. CT will show subarachnoid blood in 98% of cases within 48 hours.
• Infarction.

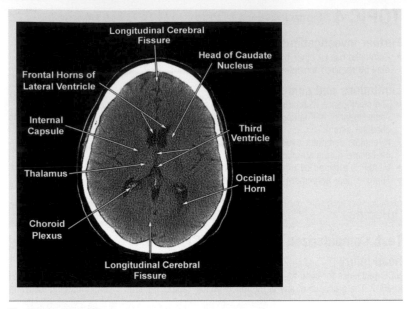

Fig. 4.5 A normal CT scan.

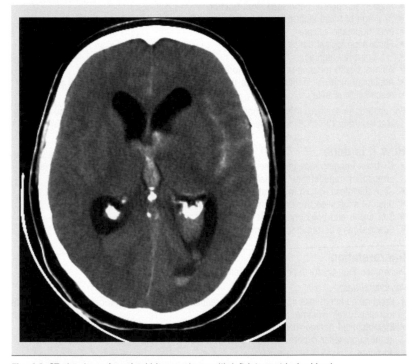

Fig. 4.6 CT showing subarachnoid haemorrhage with left intraventricular blood.

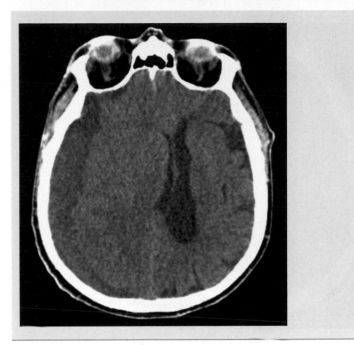

Figure 4.7 CT showing extensive right subdural haematoma with ventricular compression and midline leftward shift.

- Subdural haematoma (Fig. 4.7): initially the hyperdense space-occupying lesion gradually organizes to become hypodense, which may be difficult to differentiate from surrounding brain tissue. Check for sulcal effacement and mass effect. Compared to an extradural (which looks biconvex; lens shaped) a subdural often has a crescent-shaped appearance.
- Extradural haematoma (Fig. 4.8): due to arterial injury and skull fracture. Requires urgent neurosurgical decompression.
- Skull fractures: bone windows are required to view the cranium.
- Contusions: small areas of hyperdensity in brain substance.
- Hydrocephalus: pathological enlargement of ventricular system (Fig. 4.9).

Test: MRI brain

Advantages
- Smaller tumours are easier to see.
- MRI may detect and localize cerebral infarction within a few hours when the CT is negative.

Indications
- Better imaging of posterior aspects of brain, cerebellum and brainstem, the pituitary and parenchymal brain tissue

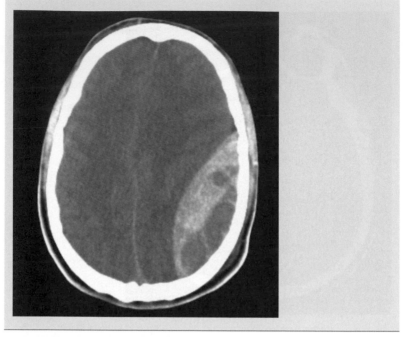

Fig. 4.8 CT showing left extradural haematoma: a biconvex (lens shaped) collection with high attenuation.

- Evaluation of brainstem, lacunar and deep white matter infarcts.
- Subtle mass effects and information re chronicity of haemorrhage.
- Evaluation of some infectious processes.
- Primary tumours (glioblastoma, astrocytoma, lymphoma) and spinal cord tumours.
- Detection and progression of CNS demyelination.
- Structural abnormalities including syringomyelia, Chiari malformations and vascular malformations.

Contraindications
Always check with radiology staff as some devices may be MRI compatible. The interference produced with metal implants may produce poor-quality pictures.

Limitations and complications
- Enclosed cylindrical magnet may precipitate claustrophobia.
- Prolonged times required for scanning.
- MRI may miss calcification.
- Specialized equipment for administration of anaesthesia and monitoring.

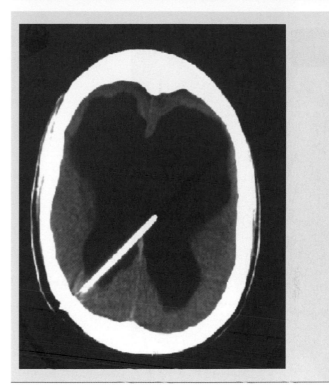

Fig. 4.9 CT showing pathological enlargement of the ventricular system and intraventricular drain.

Cervical spine in trauma

Injuries to the cervical spine occur in approximately 2–6% of blunt trauma patients, and in 10% of patients with severe head injuries with a GCS <8.

Indications

Multiple guidelines exist to suggest which patients require investigations.
- Patients who are alert and orientated, have never lost consciousness, are not under the influence of alcohol or drugs, have no distracting injuries, have no cervical tenderness and no neurological findings, and are between 2 and 65 years of age do not need imaging. All others, including all patients with a GCS <15, require some form of imaging and careful clinical assessment.

Test: Plain cervical radiographs (Fig. 4.10)

The three standard cervical trauma views are the investigation of choice according to NICE guidelines (see http://www.nice.org.uk). They consist of lateral, AP and open mouth views. The sensitivity of this series ranges from 70% to 90%. In practice this is reduced as films are inadequate in up to 50% of patients. Expert interpretation is essential.

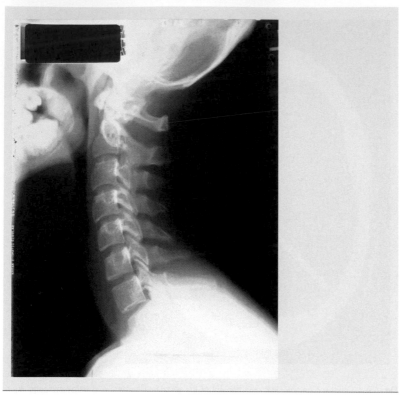

Fig. 4.10A Normal cervical spine on plain lateral radiographs.

(Continued)

How it is done

Lateral view

An adequate view from the base of the occiput to the top of T1 is mandatory. Repeated attempts to show the C7–T1 border should be avoided. Lateral views of C2 may be required to supplement CT in patients aged >65 years.

AP view

Should be correctly positioned and centered to avoid rotation artifacts and should demonstrate each spinous process from C2 to T1.

Open-mouth view

This allows visualization of the odontoid peg and the lateral masses of C1 and C2. In unconscious, head-injured patients, fractures of C1 and C2 have been missed due to obscuration by endotracheal tubes, gastric tubes and hard collars. In these intubated patients, the open-mouth view should be replaced by a CT scan.

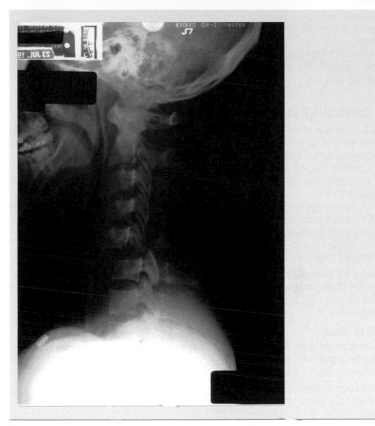

Fig. 4.10B cont'd Injured cervical spine on plain lateral radiographs.

Trauma oblique views
The trauma oblique view can indicate alignment at the C7–T1 level, if the lateral view fails to show the C7–T1 junction. It allows good visualization of the posterior elements of the cervical spine and reveals facet joint dislocations. They are not commonly undertaken in this setting in the UK.

Interpretation
Consider soft tissue and vertebral alignment. Abnormal soft tissue may be associated with a fracture and should draw attention to a hyperextension injury. Four lines can be drawn to assess alignment; disruption of any one of these smooth lines is suggestive of injury:
• Anterior margin of the vertebral bodies
• Posterior margin of the vertebral bodies
• Spinolaminar line
• Spinous processes.

Limitations

- Standard radiographs are notorious for inadequate visualization of C1/C2 and C7/T1 junctions.
- The swimmer's view requires one arm to be raised and the other pulled down, which tends to twist the spine, and dislocations have been reported. The radiation dose is also high to obtain this view.

Test: Cervical CT scan

Primary CT scanning of the entire cervical spine with sagittal and coronal reconstruction is more sensitive than plain films, particularly with the advent of the newer generation multislice/multidetector CT (MDCT) machines. Thus it has become the primary imaging of choice according to some protocols.

- NICE guidelines advocate that in patients with severe head injuries (GCS <8) CT is the imaging of choice.
- Trauma patients requiring a cranial CT should undergo either routine axial CT of C1/C2 or an MDCT examination of their entire C spine whilst still in the CT suite.
- Once one injury is detected, CT scanning of the whole cervical spine including the cervical-thoracic junction is required as 10–31% of cervical fractures have associated noncontiguous fractures.

Alternatively CT can be used as a supplement to plain films for:
- Evaluation of suspicious and poorly visualized areas
- C1 and C2 evaluation in intubated patients.

How it is done

Conventional (single slice, nonhelical) CT scanners acquire discrete axial slices. False negatives are usually due to axially orientated fractures, dislocations and undisplaced ligamentous injuries not visible with this resolution.

In a helical (spiral) scan the patient moves smoothly through the rotating scanning beam acquiring a helical volume of data, which the computer can then reconstruct in any plane.

The new MDCT machines effectively scan multiple slices simultaneously, making scanning much faster. Current recommendations for cervical spine CT are to perform 1.5–3-mm slices with reformatted sagittal and coronal reconstruction. Sagittal and coronal reconstructions must be closely examined for features suggestive of ligamentous instability, such as widening, subluxation and rotation of the vertebrae relative to one another.

The diagnostic performance of helical CT scanners is good, with reported sensitivity as high as 99% and specificity 93%. Improvements in CT technology are likely to improve sensitivity further.

Limitations

- Helical CT may not exclude unstable ligamentous injuries. Injury to the cervical spinal cord in the absence of a fracture occurs in 0.03% to 0.7% of trauma.
- It must be correctly performed and interpreted. When a fracture is not present, subtle bony malalignment and soft tissue findings may be the only clues to the presence of a potentially serious, unstable injury.
- In children under 10 years, CT of the cervical spine should only be used in cases where patients have a severe head injury (GCS ≤8), or where there is a strong suspicion of injury despite normal or inadequate plain films.

Test: Cervical MRI

Cervical MRI can detect soft tissue, ligament, disc and cord injury that may not be evident even on helical or multislice CT. To date no prospective studies comparing modern multislice CT and MRI have been conducted for the evaluation of occult cervical injuries in unconscious patients.

Indications
• Patients with neurological symptoms and signs suggesting cord or nerve root injury.

Limitations
• The requirement for detailed patient history to exclude ferrous body implants.
• Increased cervical clearance times and availability of MRI scanning.
• Risks associated with the transport of an unconscious patient, requirement of MRI-compatible monitoring equipment and prolonged scanning times.
• The incidence of soft tissue abnormalities on MRI is in the order of 20%, the significance of which is uncertain and does not correlate with other evidence of cervical instability.

Flexion/extension screening
Given the inherent risks in passively flexing and extending the neck of an unconscious patient, this technique should only be undertaken as part of a controlled trial designed to investigate efficacy and safety.

Further management principles
• In critically injured patients, spinal immobilization in hard collars and strapping can lead to decubitus ulceration, compression of the jugular veins, make airway management more difficult, restrict physiotherapy and compromise nursing care and the management of traumatic brain injury.
• Continuous spinal immobilization is therefore not recommended for >48 hours in the unconscious patient.
• To complete spinal clearance in the unconscious trauma patient ideally a CT of the whole cervical spine is obtained and reported by an expert.
• If unstable then await instructions from a spinal team.
• If normal then the hard collar can be removed. There is no need for further log rolling, but a soft Miami J collar is used for waking. When awake the neck is further tested for tenderness or pain.
• Any unexplained limb deficits require an MRI as soon as clinically possible.

Intracranial pressure (ICP) monitoring

Indications
An ICP monitor is used in traumatic brain injury when the following apply:
• Severe head injury defined as GCS <8, with an abnormal admission CT scan.
• Severe head injury with GCS <8, with a normal CT scan if two or more of the following features are present: age >40 years, unilateral or bilateral motor posturing and systolic blood pressure <90 mmHg.
• Traumatic mass lesions in selected patients with mild or moderate head injury.

Further indications for ICP monitoring are listed in Table 4.9.

Table 4.9 **Reasons for ICP monitoring**

Condition	Comments
Subarachnoid haemorrhage	With associated hydrocephalus to allow CSF drainage
Brain tumours	Selected patients at high risk of post op cerebral oedema, e.g. posterior fossa craniotomy
Reye's syndrome	Active treatment decreases mortality
Hydrocephalus	Diagnostic tool in complex cases
Benign intracranial hypertension	Monitoring via lumbar drain as diagnostic test and treatment response
Hypoxic brain swelling	Post drowning, CO poisoning
Others	Meningitis, venous sinus thrombosis, hepatic encephalopathy, stroke and craniostenosis

How it is done

Monitoring requires an invasive transducer. Ventricular drainage catheters are the gold standard. A simple catheter is inserted under sterile conditions into a lateral ventricle via a burr hole. When connected to an external pressure transducer this is the most accurate, low cost and reliable method. ICP can be controlled by CSF drainage, and the transducer may be zeroed externally.

The other commonly used method is an intraparenchymal monitor that is zeroed to atmospheric pressure before insertion.

Subdural and subarachnoid bolts are less invasive and have reduced risk of complications, but are less reliable.

Interpretation

Waveform analysis over 30 minutes should be the minimum as instant CSF measurements may be misleading. Normal range varies with age, posture and clinical conditions. Values in children are not well established (Table 4.10).

Physiological principles

The Munro Kelly hypothesis states that within the rigid skull the contents are not compressible. Initially intracranial compliance allows compensation for small increases in volume (Fig. 4.11). Once this is exhausted then small increases in volume will cause steep exponential increases in ICP.

Table 4.10 **Waveform analysis normal ranges**

Age group	Normal range (mmHg)
Adults	<10–15
Children	3–7
Term infants	1.5–6

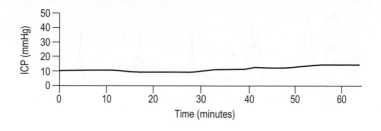

Fig. 4.11 Data presented as pressure values and/or pressure waveform against time.

Abnormalities

- Lundberg A (plateau) waves (Fig. 4.12). Steep increases in ICP from near normal values to 50–100 mmHg, persisting for 5–20 minutes and then fall sharply. Always pathological and indicate greatly reduced compliance. Often accompanied by neurological deterioration.
- Lundberg B waves (Fig. 4.13). Rhythmic oscillations occurring every 1–2 minutes. Sharp rhythmic oscillations, occurring every 1–2 minutes, occur in ventilated patients and with Cheyne–Stokes respiration. Indicative of failing intracranial compensation.

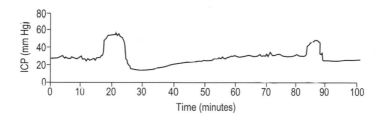

Fig. 4.12 Lundberg A waves.

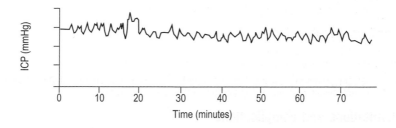

Fig. 4.13 Lundberg B Waves.

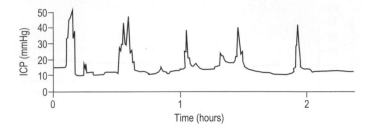

Fig. 4.14 Waves due to, for example, sudden increases in systemic blood pressure.

- Lundberg C waves. Oscillations with a frequency of 4–8/minute. They are of smaller amplitude and are probably of limited pathological significance.
- Others, for example, due to sudden increases in systemic blood pressure (Fig. 4.14).

Management principles

- Thresholds for initiating treatment vary according to aetiology.
- Brain Trauma Foundation guidelines advise that ICP treatment should be initiated at an upper threshold of 20–25 mmHg.
- Simple manoeuvres to reduce ICP include: head up tilt 15–30 degrees, unobstructed venous drainage (by not tying ET tubes and avoiding internal jugular lines), avoidance of hypoxia, maintenance of normothermia and control of PCO_2 to low normal values.
- Further management should follow protocol-driven intensive care management strategies and will include the following:
  - Analgesia and sedation
  - Neuromuscular blockade
  - Cooling to 35°C
  - Barbiturate coma
  - Osmotic diuretics (mannitol or hypertonic saline).
- For intractable intracranial hypertension measures such as CSF drainage and a decompressive craniotomy/craniectomy may be considered. A randomized controlled trial is currently evaluating use of the decompressive craniotomy.

Further investigations

- Repeat CT scans often needed.
- Additional information derived from the ICP waveforms include:
  - Cerebral perfusion pressure (CPP) (where CPP = mean arterial pressure (MAP) – (ICP + central venous pressure (CVP))) and thus CPP directed therapy.

Limitations and complications

- Overall complication rate 4–11%, including infection, haemorrhage, seizures.
- Regular calibration and patency tests required.
- Measured pressure may be compartmentalized and not necessarily representative of global ICP.

Malignant hyperthermia susceptibility

Malignant hyperthermia (MH) is a hypermetabolic condition that results from exposure to inhalational anaesthetics or suxamethonium. Abnormalities in excitation–contraction coupling cause loss of control of calcium movements, which may in turn cause a hypermetabolic response. The prevalence is estimated at 1 in 8500.

Indications for testing

- Patients in whom a suspicious MH event has occurred after exposure to known anaesthetic triggering agents. A clinical grading scale is used to assess the likelihood, which incorporates evidence of muscle rigidity, muscle breakdown, respiratory acidosis, temperature increase, cardiac involvement and family history.
- Family members of an index case.
- All patients with central core disease (CCD).
- Other possibly related diseases include Duchenne muscular dystrophy, King-Denborough syndrome, Myoadenylate deaminase deficiency and other myopathies.
- Patients with a history of exertional heat stroke or exercise-induced rhabdomyolysis, especially more than one episode.

How it is done

- Referral to the British (http://www.bmha.co.uk), nearest European (http://www.emhg.org) or North American (http://www.mhaus.org) organizations for malignant hyperthermia is required.
- The gold standard for the diagnosis of MH is the In Vitro Contracture Test (IVCT) with caffeine and halothane.
- The standardized European protocol was published in 1984: sensitivity 99% and specificity 94% have been quoted.

Interpretation

Patients are classified according to the *in vitro* contracture of the muscle tissue:
- MH susceptible (MHS) group
- MH normal (MHN) group
- MH equivocal (MHE) group.

The term MHE should be used to describe any patient with an equivocal result, regardless of family background. Some MHE patients may be clinically regarded as MH susceptible. MHE patients are considered to be under permanent review pending the acquisition of further data.

Management principles

- For emergency management of MH refer to Association of Anaesthetists of Great Britain and Ireland (AAGBI) guidelines at http://www.aagbi.org/publications/guidelines/docs/malignanthyp07.pdf.
- For future anaesthetic management avoidance of known triggering agents is paramount.
- Patient information can be found at http://www.bmha.co.uk.

Further investigations

Muscle histology
It is important that microscopic examination of the biopsy specimen occurs to detect structural abnormalities such as central core syndrome or muscular dystrophy.

Genetic testing
On confirmation of a positive index case, then referral of family members for genetic analysis is appropriate. Mutations of the ryanodine receptor type 1 (RYR1) gene have been discovered

in up to 80% of cases. The gene is large, confers autosomal dominant inheritance and is located on chromosome 19 q. Identification of all mutations is difficult due to the considerable locus and allelic heterogeneity.

The present discrepancy between genotype and phenotype should be improved by newer molecular methods to systematically identify novel mutations on the appropriate genes.

Guidelines continue to advise that patients with a negative genetic test should still undergo an IVCT to confirm phenotype and maintain patient safety.

Serum creatinine kinase (CK)
Baseline CK is increased in 50% of MH patients (Box 4.1).

Future developments
Ryanodine and chlorocresol also induce *in vitro* muscle contractures, which distinguish MH-susceptible from normal muscle. The European Malignant Hyperthermia Group have published a protocol for the use of ryanodine. Multicentre evaluation of a chlorocresol protocol is in progress.

Nuclear magnetic resonance spectroscopy is being investigated to identify MHS individuals on the basis of ATP and creatinine phosphate breakdown during graded exercise.

B lymphocytes are also being investigated as they demonstrate abnormally enhanced calcium release when stimulated with caffeine.

Limitations and complications
- The European protocol produces a group of 10–15% of patients who cannot conclusively be diagnosed either with MHS or MHN. These are termed equivocal and need further follow up.
- False positive rate of 6% using European IVCT protocol.
- Reported discordance between IVCT and genetic data in MH families. This is due to false positive/negative test results, the variable penetrance of mutations and additional factors involved in phenotype determination.

Box 4.1 **Causes of increased CK**
• Hypothyroid
• MH susceptibility
• Post op
• Neuroleptic malignant syndromes
• Rhabdomyolysis
• Duchenne muscular dystrophy
• Exercise
• Idiopathic paroxysmal rhabdomyolysis
• Malignancy
• Haemolytic syndromes
• Myocardial infarction
• Myopathies

TOPIC ⑤

Peripheral nervous system

Topic Contents

Neuromuscular block monitor 87
Test: Train of four (TOF) stimulation 87
Investigation of suxamethonium apnoea 88
Test: Dibucaine and fluoride number 90
Test: Molecular genetic testing 91
Myasthenia gravis (MG) testing 92
Test: Edrophonium (tensilon) test 92
Test: Serum anti-acetylcholinesterase receptor antibody test 92

Test: Repetitive nerve stimulation (RNS) 92
Test: Single fibre electromyography (EMG) 93
Peripheral motor and nerve function assessment 94
Test: Nerve conduction studies and electromyography (EMG) 94

Neuromuscular block monitor

Test: Train of four (TOF) stimulation

Indications

Owig to the variable individual response and a narrow therapeutic window of muscle relaxants, a peripheral nerve stimulation test is recommended after their use. In particular.

- After long-acting neuromuscular block (NMB) drugs and prolonged infusions
- Pulmonary disease, obesity and neuromuscular disorders such as myasthenia gravis and Eaton-Lambert syndrome, myopathies
- When reversal agents are contraindicated, e.g. tachyarrythmias, liver and renal dysfunction.

How it is done

- Application of a supramaximal stimulus to a peripheral nerve, followed by measurement of the associated muscular response.
- The nerve stimulator device should generate a monophasic square wave constant current up to 80 mA, and last between 0.1 and 0.5 ms.
- The nerve chosen must be close to the skin, have a motor element and muscular contraction must be visible or accessible to monitoring.
- The negative electrode should be placed directly over the superficial part of the nerve and positive electrode placed proximally to avoid direct muscular stimulation.
- The generation of single, train of four, double burst and 50-Hz patterns of stimulation is necessary. Polarity of output should be marked, and battery powered for safety.

- Small surface electrodes are used to apply to overlying skin. Good electrical contact is essential.
- Monitoring in clinical practice is by visual and tactile responses.

Interpretation

- Different patterns of nerve stimulation are used to determine onset, offset and percentage of NMB.
- Relationship between receptor occupancy and evoked responses can be estimated.

Management principles

- Onset and offset of NMB is faster in central muscles with a good blood supply.
- The most accurate muscle to monitor during NMB onset and maintenance is the orbiclaris oculi as it will reflect the conditions of the central larynx and diaphragm muscles.
- It is best to monitor a peripheral muscle such as adductor pollicis during reversal as it has a longer recovery time than respiratory muscles and will provide a greater margin of safety.
- TOF ratio >0.9 correlates with the ability to protect the airway and swallow normally. However up to 75% of receptors still remain occupied at this point.
- Clinically significant residual paralysis is defined as TOF ratio <0.9.

Stimulus responses and abnormalities
See Table 5.1.

Physiological principles

Limitations and complications

- Visual and tactile evaluation of muscular contractile response is unreliable. More accurate methods include mechanomyography (MMG), electromyography (EMG) and accelerometry (AMG) but they remain research tools.
- When monitoring is not performed up to 45% of patients are inadequately reversed on arrival to recovery room.
- When the T4–T1 ratio is 1 up to 50% of receptors can remain occupied (Table 5.2).
- Because of wide individual variability in responses, some patients may exhibit weakness at a TOF ratio of 0.8–0.9.
- Hypothermia increases skin impedance thus interpretation of evoked responses may be misleading.

Investigation of suxamethonium apnoea

Suxamethonium is metabolized by the enzyme plasma cholinesterase (ChE). Abnormalities of this enzyme may cause prolonged muscular paralysis of variable duration after suxamethonium administration. The high prevalence of variant ChE genes in the population may contribute to the measured variability in recovery time after suxamethonium administration.

The clinical picture can be caused by (Table 5.3):
- Abnormal enzyme structure and activity
- Altered plasma enzyme concentration.

Table 5.1 TOF stimulation responses

	Single twitch	Train of four (TOF)	Tetanic stimulation	Post-tetanic count	Double burst stimulation
Stimulus characteristic	Single square wave, 0.2 ms duration	4 single square stimuli at 2 Hz	50–200 Hz stimulus frequency for 5 s	A tetanic stimulus followed 3 s later by single stimuli at 1 Hz	2 short bursts 750 ms apart. Each burst has 3 stimuli, of 0.2 ms, delivered every 20 ms
Normal muscle response	Maximal muscle twitch	4 twitches of equal and maximal size	Maintained tetanic contraction. Painful	Maximal single twitches post tetany	2 contractions of equal intensity
Muscle response after NMB	Twitch depressed when NMB occupies >75% Ach receptors	Twitches fade at onset, and return during recovery after nondepolarizing block	Muscle shows fade as inability to maintain tetany, after NMB	Post-tetanic facilitation. Muscle responds to single stimuli after tetanus but not before	Response to 2nd stimuli is reduced. Tactile evaluation is more accurate than TOF ratio
Uses	Twitch depression indicates onset and duration of NMB	1. TOF count. Number of twitches correlate with degree of NMB 2. TOF ratio. Comparison of T4 to T1 correlates with degree of NMB	Monitor minor degrees of NMB	1. To assess degree of profound NMB 2. Indicates when recovery of TOF will occur	DBS ratio. Ratio of 1st:2nd stimulus is easier to assess clinically than TOF
Limitations	Least reliable. Use >10 s apart	No fade occurs during depolarizing block	Muscular fatigue may develop at frequencies 100–200 Hz in normal muscles. Use >5 min apart	Do not repeat <5 min apart	

Table 5.2 **Receptor occupancy and TOF responses after neuromuscular paralysis**

% receptors blocked	T1 % normal	T4 % normal	T4/T1 ratio	Tetanus
100				
95				
	0		T1 lost	
90	10		T2 lost	
	20		T3 lost	
80	25	0	T4 lost	Onset of fade at 30 Hz
	80–90	55–65	0.6–0.7	
	95	70	0.7–0.75	
75	100	75–100	0.75–1	
	100		0.9–1	Onset of fade at 50 Hz
50				Onset of fade at 100 Hz
30				Onset of fade at 200 Hz

Table 5.3 **Causes of suxamethonium apnoea**

Genetic variants	Acquired causes
Atypical A	Pregnancy
Fluoride resistant F	Liver disease
Silent S	Carcinomatosis
H (10% reduced concentration)	Cardiac failure
J (33% reduced concentration)	Uraemia
K (66% reduced concentration)	Myxoedema
	Burns
	Poor nutrition
	Drugs: procaine, lithium, magnesium, ketamine, OCP, ecothiopate, tacrine

OCP, Oral Contraceptive Pill

Test: Dibucaine and fluoride number

Indications
- Prolonged apnoea (muscle relaxation) post suxamethonium or mivacurium administration as detected by a neuromuscular TOF monitor.

How it is done
Biochemical measurement of ChE activity with inhibitors is a standard method of measurement. Testing must not occur within 24 hours of drug administration.

Dibucaine number
- Normal plasma ChE is inhibited by dibucaine.
- Plasma is added to benzylcholine and the light emitted is detected by a spectrophotometer.
- This is then repeated with plasma plus 10^{-5} M dibucaine.
- Percentage inhibition of benzylcholine broken down by the ChE is measured as the dibucaine number.

Flouride number
- The fluoride-resistant plasma's ChE enzyme variant is similarly identified by its percent inhibition of benzylcholine hydrolysis when fluoride is added to the assay.

Interpretation

Data presented as
- Dibucaine number and fluoride number (Table 5.4).

Table 5.4 **Common cholinesterase genotypes and their effect upon dibucaine number, fluoride number and phenotype**

Commonest genotypes	Population incidence (%)	Dibucaine number	Fluoride number	Duration of post-suxamethonium apnoea
E1uE1u	94	75–85	>60	5 min
E1fE1f	0.003	70	<30	1 h
E1aE1a	0.03	20	20	1–2 h
E1sE1s	0.001	0	0	>3 h
E1uE1f	0.5	75	50	10 min
E1uE1a	3	50	45	10 min
E1uE1s	0.5	80	60	10 min

Limitations
- Biochemical tests are a measure of phenotype. This does not allow accurate determination of underlying genotype.
- They cannot distinguish between primary and secondary deficiencies.
- The duration of neuromuscular block can be different with patients of identical genotypes.
- Biochemical test results may remain normal in the presence of some clinically affected variants.
- ChE activity is higher in small children than adults and results have to be analyzed according to age.
- Heterozygotes are usually clinically insignificant unless accompanied by another mutation or an acquired cause of plasma ChE deficiency.

Test: Molecular genetic testing
- The gene that codes for the ChE enzyme is located at the E1 locus on the long arm of chromosome 3.

- More than 20 mutations have been identified in the plasma cholinesterase gene. They include: normal plasma ChE (u); atypical hydrolyzing activity (a), fluoride resistant (f), silent (s).
- Some mutations code for decreased concentration with normal activity: H, J and K variants.
- One further rare variant allele is C5, which has higher than normal ChE activity. It manifests as suxamethonium resistance.
- Genes follow typical autosomal recessive inheritance, and some by linkage disequilibrium.

Myasthenia gravis (MG) testing

Myasthenia gravis (MG) is an autoimmune disease of the neuromuscular junction (NMJ) characterized by fatigable muscle weakness. It has an incidence of 1 in 100 000; average age of onset 20–30 years in women and 40–50 years in men.

Indications

- The diagnosis is based upon a characteristic history and examination, positive serological and electrophysiological diagnostic tests.
- The characteristic history is of weakness and/or fatigue in the voluntary muscles, increasing during the course of the day, worsening after exertion and improving with rest. It may involve ocular muscles only.

Test: Edrophonium (tensilon) test

- The tensilon (edrophonium) test can be performed at the bedside, but is neither sensitive nor specific for MG. It should only be performed when the diagnosis is required urgently. Full cardiac monitoring and atropine is required in case of cardiovascular side effects. Initially 2 mg (max 10 mg) edrophonium is administered IV.
- Edrophonium inhibits acetylcholinesterase (ACh) and prolongs the duration of ACh available at the neuromuscular junction (NMJ).
- A response is usually seen within a few minutes. An objective improvement in muscle strength is noted in a positive test.

Test: Serum anti-acetylcholinesterase receptor antibody test
How it is done
- Serum is taken for measurement of the IgG and IgM anti-ACh receptor antibodies.

Interpretation
- Anti-ACh receptor antibodies are positive in 85–90% adult MG, 50% childhood MG, 60% ocular MG and 100% associated with thymoma.
- Titres do not correspond to severity.
- False positives occur with penicillamine, immune liver disorders, Lambert-Eaton syndrome (13%), lung cancer and the elderly (>70 years).

Test: Repetitive nerve stimulation (RNS)
How it is done
- The nerve supplying an affected muscle is stimulated 6–10 times at 2–3 Hz.
- Using surface electrodes over the muscle a compound motor action potential (CMAP) is recorded.

Interpretation
Data is presented as a compound motor action potential (CMAP) (Fig. 5.1).

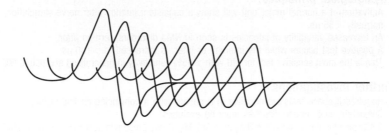

Fig. 5.1 Compound motor action potential (CMAP) from a muscle showing the progressive reduction in amplitude seen with repetitive stimulation.

Physiological principles
- In normal muscles there is no change with repetitive stimulation.
- CMAP amplitude decreases by greater than 10% in a positive test.
- The decrement is often enhanced following exercise.
- RNS decrement is seen in 75% of generalized MG, 50% ocular MG.
- A decremental response alone is not specific for MG and can be seen in other motor neuron disorders.

Test: Single fibre EMG
How it is done
- Undertaken in equivocal patients.
- The muscle fibre potentials from the same motor unit are monitored after a single axon innervation.

Interpretation
See Fig. 5.2.

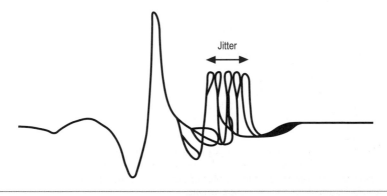

Fig. 5.2 Seven discharges superimposed to show variability in time interval caused by insecure neuromuscular junction transmission.

Physiological principles

- Activation of a normal motor unit will show a consistent latency after nerve stimulation, normally <55 μs.
- An increased variability of latencies is seen in NMJ disorders, termed *jitter*.
- A positive test occurs when the interval, or jitter, is increased to >100 μs.
- This is the most sensitive test for MG with $>95\%$ sensitivity in generalized and ocular MG.

Further investigations

- Required if above tests are negative in a patient with a convincing clinical history.
- Coexistent autoimmune diseases must be excluded.
- Antibodies to other areas of the NMJ (e.g. Anti MuSK) are present in 50% of seronegative MG.
- Muscle biopsy can be useful.
- CT/MRI thorax is necessary for diagnosis of thymomas and thymic hyperplasia.
- MRI of the brain may be necessary if a structural brain lesion is suspected.
- Exclude underlying malignancy.

Peripheral motor and nerve function assessment

Test: Nerve conduction studies and electromyography (EMG)

To evaluate the integrity and function of the peripheral nervous system.

Indications

Diagnosis and assessment of the following:

- Neuropathy – metabolic (diabetes mellitus, uraemia, hypothyroid, hepatic, HIV immune causes, rheumatoid arthritis, systemic lupus erythematosus), traumatic, entrapment, idiopathic mononeuropathies, clinical suspicion of amyotrophic lateral sclerosis (ALS), inflammatory (e.g. post polio, Guillain Barré syndrome), hereditary (e.g. Charcot Marie Tooth)
- Myopathy – Hereditary or inflammatory (e.g. polymyositis, critical illness myopathy)
- Neuromuscular junction – myasthenia gravis, Eaton-Lambert syndrome.

Perioperative monitoring:

- Facial nerve monitoring during posterior fossa neurosurgery and middle ear surgery
- Spinal surgery: during cauda equina surgery the anal sphincter and leg muscles can be monitored.

How it is done

- The selected nerve is stimulated using a current that will excite all the axons in the nerve trunk. The electric output is a rectangular wave, duration 0.1–0.2 ms. Needle electrodes may be required when stimulating a deep nerve. Stimulation should be performed at two or more sites along the nerve.
- Propagated activity is recorded at a distance along the nerve or from the muscle using a surface or needle recording electrode. The muscle response after nerve stimulation is the compound muscle action potential (CMAP).

Interpretation

Data presented as:

- Latency. The time between stimulus and response includes nerve conduction time and neuromuscular transmission time.
- Amplitude. This depends upon the number of axons that conduct impulses, the number of functioning endplates and the muscle volume.
- Conduction velocity (CV). Normally 40–60 m/s

Abnormalities

Pathological findings include conduction slowing, conduction block, no response, low amplitude response. This can evaluate the degree of demyelination and axonal loss in nerves studied.

- Demyelination: reduces maximal CV and may produce conduction block.
- Axonal loss: small action potentials (amplitude) with normal CV.
- In normal muscle no electrical activity occurs at rest, motor neurons discharge on voluntary contraction, and responses can be recorded. (MUAP).
- Degeneration of motor neurons results in small potentials recorded from muscles at rest: fibrillations and positive sharp waves, and the number of motor units on contraction decreases.
- Myopathic muscle becomes wasted and fibres shrink, MUAPs are smaller than normal, contraction is weak despite normal motor conduction. Sometimes needle insertion itself provokes bursts of muscle APs.

Management principles

- Neurophysiological data strongly suggests that critical illness myopathy is more common than previously assumed.
- Electrophysiological measurements can be obtained from the phrenic nerve and diaphragm in cases of respiratory weaning failure.

Further investigations

- Single fibre Electromyography.
- Quantitative EMG, direct muscle stimulation and other detailed assessments.

Limitations and complications

- Neurogenic and myopathic weakness can be difficult to distinguish clinically.
- Absence of a sensory nerve AP may be due to Na channel dysfunction, not necessarily peripheral nerve degeneration.
- It is difficult to distinguish different neuromuscular disorders in the critically ill as they are unable to cooperate with testing. Referral to expert centres is recommended.

Local oedema, electronic devices, lines and monitors frequently prevents reliable sensory recordings in intensive care.

TOPIC 6

Renal, metabolic and endocrine systems

Topic Contents

Assessment of renal function:
Serological tests 97
Test: Serum creatinine 97
Test: Serum urea measurement 100
Assessment of renal function:
urinalysis 101
Test: Urine dipstick 101
Test: Urine microscopy 101
Test: Laboratory assay of urine sodium,
osmolality, urea, creatinine and
specific gravity 102
Assessment of renal function:
Measurement of glomerular filtration
rate 104
Test: Radioisotope assay 104
Test: Inulin clearance 105
Test: Creatinine clearance 105
Assessment of renal function:
Radiological 106
Test: Renal ultrasound 106
Serological measurement of
electrolytes 107
Test: Serum sodium measurement 107
Test: Serum potassium measurement 109
Test: Serum magnesium 112
Test: Serum calcium 113
Test: Serum phosphate 115
Test: Serum chloride 117

Test: Serum lactate 117
Test: Serum bicarbonate 118
Investigation of salt and water
disturbance 119
Test: Serum osmolality 119
Assessment of thyroid function 120
Test: Serum thyroid hormones
measurement 120
Assessment of glycaemic control 121
Test: Serum glucose 121
Test: Glycosylated haemoglobin
(HbA1C) 124
Investigation of the
hypothalamic–pituitary axis 124
Test: Short synacthen test 124
Measurement of hormones:
Phaeochromocytoma 125
Test: Plasma and urine catecholamines and
their metabolites 125
Measurement of hormones: Carcinoid
tumours 127
Test: Urinary 5-hydroxyindole acetic acid
(5-HIAA) 127
Investigation of allergic reactions 127
Test: Serum mast cell tryptase
measurement 127
Test: Serum and urine histamine assay 128

Assessment of renal function: Serological tests

Test: Serum creatinine

Indications
1. Assessment of renal function.
2. Suspected or proven rhabdomyolysis.
3. As part of routine preoperative assessment for certain patients/procedures (see NICE guidelines available at http://www.nice.org.uk/CG003).

Data presented as
Numerical value: units (μmol/L).

Interpretation
Physiological principles
- Creatinine is a basic compound that is formed mainly in skeletal muscle from phosphorylcreatine.
- Except in rhabdomyolysis, production of creatinine is fairly constant; thus creatinine levels in the serum are a useful reflection of renal function as its elimination is entirely renal.

Normal range
- 60–130 μmol/L. Normal values vary according to gender and ethnic origin.

Abnormalities and management principles
- Serum creatinine increases slowly with a reduction in glomerular filtration rate (GFR) down to 40 mL/min; thereafter, creatinine rises sharply with small reductions in GFR, reducing its usefulness as a measure of renal function at high values (Fig. 6.1).

Renal failure/impairment
- Renal failure may be acute or chronic. Identification of the cause of renal failure can only be achieved using a combination of history taking and clinical evaluation, in conjunction with further investigations.
- The RIFLE criteria (Fig. 6.2) are an evidence-based guide to aid classification of the degree of renal dysfunction, based on serum creatinine and urine output.

The acronym RIFLE encompasses three levels of renal dysfunction ('risk of renal dysfunction', 'injury to kidney' and 'failure of renal dysfunction') and two outcomes of renal dysfunction ('loss' and 'end-stage renal disease'). The inclusion of these two separate outcomes acknowledges the important adaptations that occur in end-stage renal disease (ESRD) that are not seen in persistent acute renal failure (ARF). Persistent ARF (loss) is defined as need for renal replacement therapy (RRT) for more than 4 weeks, whereas ESRD is defined by need for dialysis for longer than 3 months.

Acute renal failure
See Table 6.1 for causes.
Prerenal uraemia versus acute tubular necrosis
- Both caused by renal hypoperfusion and ischaemia.
- In prerenal uraemia, renal function is salvageable with restoration of perfusion; in ATN, disruption of physiological mechanisms such as the renin-angiotensin system necessitate renal replacement therapy.
Management principles
- Identification and management of underlying cause.
- Treatment of fluid overload, acidosis and hyperkalaemia, using renal replacement therapy if required.

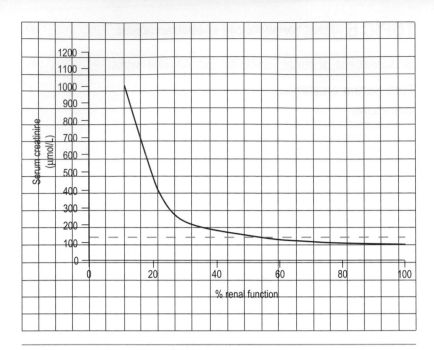

Fig. 6.1 Serum creatinine versus renal function.

	GFR criteria	Urine output (UO) criteria	
Risk	Increased SCreat × 1.5 or GFR decrease > 25%	UO < 0.5mL/kg/h x 6 h	High sensitivity
Injury	Increased SCreat × 2 or GFR decrease > 50%	UO < 5mL/kg/h × 12 h	
Failure	Increased SCreat × 3 GFR decrease 75% OR SCreat ≥ 4mg/dL Acute rise ≥ 0.5mg/dL	UO < 0.3mL/kg/h × 24 hr or anuria × 12 h	Oliguria — High specificity
Loss	Persistent ARF = complete loss of kidney function > 4 weeks		
ESKD	End-stage kidney disease (> 3 months)		

Fig. 6.2 The RIFLE criteria for classification of renal dysfunction. (Adapted from Bellomo et al. (2004) Crit Care Med 8:R204-R212, with permission.)

Table 6.1 Causes and classifications of acute renal failure

Classification		Example of causes
'Pre-renal'	Pre-renal failure causing renal hypoperfusion and acute tubular necrosis	Circulating volume depletion: dehydration, haemorrhage, etc Low cardiac output of any origin Sepsis Drugs causing reduction in renal perfusion (e.g. NSAIDs, ACE inhibitors)
'Intrinsic renal'	Acute glomerulonephritis and vasculitis	ANCA-positive vasculitis (e.g. Wegener's) Goodpasture's disease Systemic lupus erythematosus Endocarditis
	Disruption of renal vasculature	Large vessel occlusion (renovascular disease) Small vessel occlusion (DIC, haemolytic-uraemic syndrome; thrombotic thrombocytopenic purpura; pre-eclampsia)
	Toxic acute tubular necrosis	Drugs (e.g. gentamicin) Contrast nephropathy Myoglobinuria from rhabdomyolysis
	Interstitial nephritis	Idiopathic/autoimmune Drug-induced hypersensitivity Infection
	Myeloma/tubular cast nephropathy	
'Post-renal' or 'obstructive'	Urinary tract obstruction	Prostatic disease; renal stones

Chronic renal failure
See Table 6.2 for causes.

Other causes of a raised creatinine, without a concomitant rise in urea
- Drugs: cimetidine, trimethroprim, aspirin.
- Other: liver failure, racial variations, rhabdomyolysis (before onset of associated renal failure).

Management principles
- Identification and treatment of underlying aetiology.
- Renal replacement therapy with dialysis or transplantation when end-stage renal failure reached.

Limitations and complications
There is considerable inter-individual variation in normal serum creatinine due to muscle mass, age and diet. Thus, only serial measurements will provide a useful indication of changes in renal function.

Table 6.2 **Causes of chronic renal failure**	
Intrinsic causes	**Obstructive causes**
Diabetic nephropathy	Post-obstructive nephropathy
Chronic glomerulonephritis	Nephrolithiasis
Renovascular disease	Multiple myeloma
Chronic reflux nephropathy	
Polycystic kidney disease	
Amyloidosis	
Post-acute renal failure	
Chronic interstitial nephritis	
Analgesic nephropathy	

Test: Serum urea measurement

Indications
1. Investigation of renal function.
2. As part of routine preoperative assessment for certain patients/procedures (see NICE guidelines).

Data presented as
Numerical value: units mmol/L.

Interpretation
Physiological principles
- Urea (NH_2CONH_2) is a product of the hepatic metabolism of amino acids, produced from the hydrolysis of arginine in the urea cycle.
- It is freely filtered by the glomerulus; approximately 50% is subsequently reabsorbed in the proximal tubule and contributes to the counter-current exchange mechanism.
- The remainder is excreted in the urine, accounting for over 80% of the body's daily nitrogen excretion.

Normal range
2.5–7.0 mmol/L.

Abnormalities
- In most cases, an elevated urea (>12 mmol/L) represents impairment of renal function and is accompanied by a concomitant increase in serum creatinine.
- In some situations, serum urea may rise out of proportion with serum creatinine:
1. Prerenal failure (e.g. due to dehydration, heart failure, renal artery stenosis)
2. Gastrointestinal bleeding (protein meal)
3. High dietary protein intake
4. Steroids
5. Old tetracycline ingestion
6. Addison's disease

Management principles

See under 'Serum creatinine'.

Assessment of renal function: urinalysis

Test: urine dipstick

Indications

1. Bedside investigation of renal function.
2. Screening for diabetes.
3. Screening for urinary tract infection.

How it is done

- A reagent stick is dipped into a urine sample.
- The various reagents change colour according to the presence of various constituents of the sample.

Data presented as

Reagent stick colour changes compared to standardized colour chart.

Interpretation

Physiological principles

- If substances such as glucose, protein or red or white cells appear in the urine, this indicates either an abnormally high systemic generation of these substances, or an inability of the kidney to handle these substances normally, as may be the case with intrinsic renal disease.

Normal range

- pH <5.3.
- Specific gravity 1.002–1.005.
- Trace protein and white cells.
- Absence of glucose, ketones and red cells.
- No bilirubin; minimal urobilinogen; no nitrites.

Abnormalities and management principles

A few causes of an abnormal urine dipstick are listed in Table 6.3.

Limitations and complications

Urine dipstick is a very nonspecific test and further investigation will always be required in the presence of an abnormal result.

Test: Urine microscopy

Indications

- Investigation of abnormal renal function.
- Suspected urinary tract infection.

How it is done

Microscopic laboratory analysis of a fresh urine sample.

Table 6.3 Causes of abnormal urine dipstick

Finding	Causes
Glycosuria	Diabetes mellitus
	Tubular dysfunction
	Pregnancy
Proteinuria	Glomerular dysfunction, e.g. pre-eclamptic toxaemia
	Orthostatic proteinuria (benign; occurs after prolonged standing)
	Fever
	Severe exercise
	Lower urinary tract infection
	Nephrotic syndrome
High pH	Distal renal tubular acidosis (renal bicarbonate losses)
Low specific gravity	Diabetes insipidus
Red cells	Rhabdomyolysis
	Urinary tract infection
	Glomerulonephritis
Leucocytes	Urinary tract infection
Nitrites	Gram-negative bacterial urinary tract infection
Bilirubin/increased urobilinogen	Conjugated bilirubin appears in presence of obstructive jaundice

Data presented as

Written report detailing presence or absence of cells, crystals and casts.

Interpretation

Physiological principles

Cells, crystals and casts are not usually found in the urine and their presence may indicate the presence of intrinsic renal pathology or infection.

Abnormalities and management principles

See Table 6.4 for explanation of various findings.

Limitations and complications

Sample contamination may affect the result. This is a fairly nonspecific test, and further investigations will be required to make a diagnosis if an abnormal result is found.

Test: Laboratory assay of urine sodium, osmolality, urea, creatinine and specific gravity

Indications

Differentiation between prerenal oliguria and acute tubular necrosis.

Table 6.4 Findings in the urine on microscopy

Finding	Causes
Red cells	Glomerular bleeding or dysfunction
	Infection
	Traumatic catheterization
White cells	Infection
	Some cases of glomerular disease
	Some cases of interstitial nephritis
Crystals	Renal calculi
	Gout (uric acid crystals)
Casts	
Hyaline casts	Normal
Granular casts	Nonspecific
Tubular cell casts	Acute tubular necrosis or interstitial nephritis
Red cell casts	Glomerulonephritis or glomerular bleeding
Leucocyte casts	Acute tubular necrosis or pyelonephritis

Interpretation

Physiological principles

- In prerenal uraemia an acute hypoperfusion insult to the kidney has occurred, but there is preservation of physiological mechanisms within the kidney (such as stimulation of the renin-angiotensin-aldosterone system) which maintain normal sodium and water handling within the nephron.
- In the case of acute tubular necrosis, kidney damage has occurred, impairing normal solute and water handling; in the oliguric patient, urinalysis may differentiate between these two disorders and guide management.

Normal ranges

See Table 6.5.

Table 6.5 Normal ranges for urine laboratory findings

Investigation	Prerenal oliguria	Acute tubular necrosis
Urine sodium (mmol/L)	<20	>40
Specific gravity	>1.020	<1.010
Urine osmolality (mosmol/kg)	>500	<350
Urine: plasma osmolality ratio	>2	<1.1
Urine: plasma urea ratio	>20	<10
Urine: plasma creatinine ratio	>40	<20
Fractional sodium excretion*	<<1%	>1%

*Percentage of sodium filtered at the glomerulus (normally 1000 mmol/hour), which actually appears in the urine (normally 6 mmol/hour; i.e. 0.6%).

Abnormalities and management principles
Patients with prerenal oliguria may have their renal function salvaged by aggressive haemodynamic and fluid resuscitation. In patients with established ATN, renal replacement therapy is likely to be required.

Limitations and complications
These values will be affected by the use of diuretics. In clinical practice, it would be unusual for clinical decision making to be based on urinalysis alone.

Assessment of renal function: Measurement of glomerular filtration rate

Test: Radioisotope assay

Indications
'Gold standard' laboratory assessment of renal function.

How it is done
A precalculated dose of a radiolabelled isotope such as ^{51}chromium-EDTA or ^{99}technetium-DTPA is injected intravenously into the patient. The clearance of the isotope is calculated using the formula:

$$Clearance = dose/area\ under\ plasma\ concentration\ time\ curve$$

Data presented as
Numerical value: units mL/min.

Interpretation
Physiological principles
Glomerular filtration rate (GFR) is the volume of fluid (in mL) filtered from the renal glomerular capillaries into the Bowman's capsule per unit time (minutes). This is a measure of renal function.

The radioisotope is cleared entirely renally, thus its clearance will correlate with GFR.

Normal range
Male: 97–137 mL/minute
Female: 88–128 mL/minute

Abnormalities and management principles
Glomerular filtration rate is reduced by:
1. Any cause of renal impairment
2. Age: GFR reduces by approximately 1 mL/minute/year over the age of 30.

Glomerular filtration rate may be increased by:
1. Pregnancy
2. Exercise

Limitations and complications
- Not accurate in patients with significant oedema, as the expanded extracellular volume will influence the disappearance of the plasma tracer.

- Isotope assay is a relatively time-consuming and invasive technique. In clinical practice, creatinine clearance is usually preferred to isotope assay in the assessment of renal dysfunction.

Test: Inulin clearance

Indications

Laboratory assessment of renal function.

How it is done

Inulin, a chemically inert substance, is administered to the patient by a constant infusion and the plasma and urine concentrations measured. GFR is calculated using a variation on the clearance formula.

Physiological principles

- Measurement of glomerular filtration rate is possible by measuring the clearance of a substance that is metabolically inert, does not interfere with renal function, is neither bound nor excreted by an extrarenal route and is freely filtered by the glomerulus without being secreted or reabsorbed elsewhere in the nephron.
- Inulin fulfils all the above criteria. Prior to the development of radioisotope assays, it was used as the 'gold standard' for measuring glomerular filtration rate.

Limitations and complications

Inulin clearance is rarely used now as it has been superseded by isotope assays. It is a relatively invasive and complicated investigation, and in the bedside assessment of GFR, measurement or calculation of creatinine clearance (see below) is preferred as a simpler, less time-consuming and more practical method.

Test: Creatinine clearance

Indications

Bedside assessment of renal function.

How it is done

Creatinine clearance can be estimated using a variety of methods; three of the commonest are listed below.

1. 24-hour creatinine clearance

Laboratory assays of serum and urinary creatinine are required (see before). The creatinine clearance is then calculated using a modification of the generic equation to calculate clearance:

$$24\text{-hour creatinine clearance (mL/minute)} =$$

$$\frac{\text{urine concentration creatinine } (\mu g/mL) \times \text{urine volume (mL)}}{\text{Plasma concentration creatinine } (\mu g/mL) \times 1440 \text{ (min)}}$$

(1440 = number of minutes in 24 hours.)

2. Cockroft-Gault formula

Laboratory measurement of serum creatinine and the patient's age, sex and weight are required.

$$\text{Male GFR(mL/minute)} = \frac{(140 - \text{age}) \times \text{weight in kg}}{\text{Serum creatinine(mg/dL)} \times 72}$$

$$\text{Female GFR(mL/minute)} = \frac{(140 - \text{age}) \times \text{weight in kg} \times 0.85}{\text{Serum creatinine(mg/dL)} \times 72}$$

3. Abbreviated MDRD Study equation

MDRD is the acronym for the Modification of Diet in Renal Disease Study equation:

$$\text{GFR(mL/minute/1.73m}^2) = 186 \times \text{serum creatinine in mg/dL}^{-1.154.} \times \text{age}^{-0.203}$$

Adjustments:
- Female: multiply GFR by 0.742
- Afro-Caribbean: multiply GFR by 1.210.

Data presented as

Numerical value.

Units: mL/minute for 24 hours creatinine clearance and Cockroft-Gault and mL/minute/1.73 m^2 for abbreviated MDRD Study equation.

Interpretation

Physiological principles
- Creatinine is the naturally occurring molecule that most closely fits the above criteria.
- 24-hour creatinine clearance thus measures GFR; the Cockroft-Gault and abbreviated MDRD equations estimate creatinine clearance and thus GFR.

Normal range
1. 24-hour creatinine clearance and Cockroft-Gault formula:
   - Male: 97–137 mL/minute
   - Female: 88–128 mL/minute.
2. Abbreviated MDRD equation 75–116 mL/minute/1.73 m^2 depending on age.

Limitations and complications
- Creatinine secretion in the tubule may be a cause of a small error; not generally clinically relevant.
- Drugs that reduce tubular creatinine secretion may cause inaccuracies, e.g. cimetidine, certain antibiotics and quinidine.

Assessment of renal function: Radiological

Test: Renal ultrasound

Indications
1. Investigation of renal impairment/failure.
2. Preoperative assessment for live related kidney donors.

How it is done
Abdominal ultrasound examination.

Data presented as
Radiological imaging, with measurement of kidney size.

Interpretation

Physiological principles
- Renal size:
  - Renal length will be normal bilaterally in most causes of acute renal failure
  - The kidneys will be small bilaterally in many causes of chronic renal failure (<8 cm)
  - Asymmetrical renal size may reflect renovascular disease.
- Structural abnormalities:
  - Mass lesions such as tumours, simple cysts or polycystic kidney disease can be identified
  - Causes of postrenal obstruction such as prostatic enlargement may also be revealed
  - Calculi may be visible within the kidney or urological tract
  - Cortical scarring caused by reflux nephropathy or following segmental ischaemia will be visible.

Normal range
Bipolar renal length: 9–13 cm in adults.

Limitations and complications
- Operator dependent.
- Difficult in patients with large body habitus.

Serological measurement of electrolytes

Test: Serum sodium measurement

Indications
1. Preoperative biochemistry profile according to NICE guidelines.
2. Critical illness, renal or hepatic failure.
3. Disordered water homeostasis of any cause including suspected diabetes insipidus or syndrome of inappropriate ADH secretion (SIADH).
4. Adrenal disorders.

How it is done
Radioimmunoassay.

Interpretation

Physiological principles
- Sodium is the predominant extracellular cation and principal osmotically active solute in plasma and interstitial fluid; it is vital for membrane potentials and action potentials.
- It is actively absorbed from the small intestine and colon under the influence of aldosterone; freely filtered at the glomerulus and then actively reabsorbed in the proximal convoluted tubule, utilizing Na,K-ATPase.
- Lost predominantly in urine (150 mmol/day); some loss from sweat, faeces and saliva (10 mmol/day each).
- Sodium balance is regulated via:
  - osmoreceptors, which monitor extracellular sodium concentration then influence the renin-angiotensin-aldosterone system
  - Baroreceptors, which monitor changes in extracellular volume so influencing antidiuretic hormone and atrial natriuretic hormone secretion as well as the renin-angiotensin-aldosterone system.

Normal range
135–145 mmol/L.

Abnormalities and management principles

Hyponatraemia
Causes
Hyponatraemia may be divided into three categories:
1. 'Real' hyponatraemia (hypo-osmolar plasma)
2. Pseudo-hyponatraemia (i.e. presence of high levels of triglycerides or proteins with a normal serum osmolality)
3. Dilutional hyponatraemia: hyperosmolar plasma due to water shift from intracellular to extracellular compartments, e.g. due to the presence of ethanol, hyperglycaemia or mannitol administration.

Assessment of total body fluid status and the measurement of urinary sodium are both crucial to identifying the cause of hyponatraemia. Causes of 'real' hyponatraemia may be classified as in Table 6.6.

Table 6.6 **Causes of 'real' hyponatraemia**		
Urine sodium (mmol/L)	Eu or hypervolaemia with oedema	Hypovolaemia
>20	Renal failure SIADH Hypothyroidism Drugs with antidiuretic effect (e.g. oxytocin, chlorpropamide)	Diuretics Salt-losing nephropathy Hypoadrenalism Renal tubular acidosis Post-relief of urinary obstruction
<10	Excessive water intake: • Sodium deficient Intravenous Infusion (IVI) • Trans Urethral Resection of the Prostate (TURP) syndrome • Excessive drinking Congestive cardiac failure Liver cirrhosis Nephrotic syndrome	Diarrhoea and vomiting Acute pancreatitis Other fluid loss

Clinical features
• Depend on the underlying cause.
• In true hyponatraemia, features of dehydration and hypovolaemia predominate.
• In hypervolaemic hyponatraemia, symptoms occur with serum sodium levels of <120 mmol/L and are predominantly neurological, including headache, nausea and confusion. If untreated, this may progress to convulsions and coma.
• Osmotic intracellular movement of water may lead to permanent neurological deficit.

Management principles
• Identification and treatment of underlying cause.
• In severe cases of sodium and water deficiency, correction with hypertonic saline.
• Avoid rapid correction (risk of pontine myelinolysis, subdural haemorrhage or cardiac failure).
• Suggested correction rate: 2 mmol/L/hour until serum sodium reaches 120 mmol/L thereafter a maximum correction rate of 5–10 mmol/L/day.

- Calculation of total sodium deficit may assist in correction; assuming normal sodium distribution throughout total body water, sodium deficit may be calculated:

$$(125 - [Na^+]) \times (0.6 \times \text{body weight in kg})$$

Hypernatraemia

The causes of hypernatraemia can be classified as in Table 6.7, paying attention to the urinary sodium concentration.

Table 6.7 **Causes of hypernatraemia**	
Urine sodium	**Examples**
>20 mmol – true hypernatraemia	Iatrogenic (e.g. administration of hypertonic saline or sodium bicarbonate solutions) Cushing's syndrome Conn's syndrome (hyperaldosteronism)
<20 mmol – sodium depletion with greater water depletion	Renal loss from osmotic diuresis (e.g. hyperglycaemia, uraemia, administration of mannitol)
<10 mmol – sodium depletion with more severe water depletion	Adrenocortical insufficiency Increase in insensible losses – e.g. from sweating or suppurating wounds Diarrhoea and vomiting
Variable urinary sodium – pure water depletion	Renal water loss from diabetes insipidus Dehydration from insufficient water intake

Clinical features
- Those of dehydration, if present: thirst, and progressive neurological obtundation.
- If severe, cerebral dehydration may occur, leading to intracerebral haemorrhage from vessel disruption.

Treatment
- Identify and manage underlying cause
  - History, examination and urine sodium measurement.
  - Urine and serum cortisol measurements and plasma ACTH will reveal Cushing's syndrome.
- Rehydration with enteral water where possible; if not, use 0.9% saline IV.
- Hypotonic saline may be used in severe salt and water deficiency.
- Careful slow correction required to prevent cerebral oedema and convulsions.

Limitations and complications

Serum sodium measurement can be inaccurate in uraemia or hyperbilirubinaemia.

Test: Serum potassium measurement

Indications

1. Preoperative assessment according to NICE guidelines.
2. Renal impairment.

3. Critical illness.
4. Diuretic therapy.
5. Cardiac dysrhythmias.
6. Intravenous or enteral nutrition.

How it is done
Spectophotometric assay of serum sample.

Interpretation
Physiological principles
- Potassium is the principal intracellular cation; essential to the electrical excitability of cells and the maintenance of membrane potentials.
- It is freely filtered at the glomerulus and then reabsorbed, predominantly in the proximal convoluted tubule.
- Actively secreted in the distal tubule under the influence of aldosterone, in exchange for sodium and hydrogen ions.

Normal range
3.5–4.5 mmol/L.

Abnormalities and management principles
Hypokalaemia
Classification of the causes of hypokalaemia can be made according to the urinary potassium excretion and plasma renin activity (Table 6.8).

Table 6.8 **Causes of hypokalaemia**		
Potassium excretion <30 mmol/day	Potassium excretion >30 mmol/day with low plasma renin activity	Potassium excretion >30 mmol/day with high plasma renin activity
Gastrointestinal losses Low intake: e.g. due to parenteral fluid therapy without potassium supplementation Previous diuretic usage Movement of potassium into cells: e.g. due to alkalosis or drugs such as insulin and catecholamines	Conn's syndrome (primary hyperaldosteronism) and other disorders of the renin-angiotensin system Renal tubular acidosis Liquorice Carbenoxalone	Diuretic use Salt-wasting chronic renal failure Diuretic phase of acute renal failure Accelerated hypertension Renovascular disease Cushing's syndrome Bartter's syndrome Renin-secreting tumours

Treatment
- Replacement: either orally (up to 200 mmol/day) or intravenously (up to a maximum of 40 mmol/hour).
- Too high a concentration of intravenous potassium may cause necrosis of small veins; if significant replacement is required, a central line is recommended.
- Too rapid a correction will result in ventricular fibrillation; if quick correction is required, cardiac monitoring is indicated.

Hyperkalaemia

Causes of hyperkalaemia can be divided into those that result from increased intake, decrease output or transcellular movement into the plasma (Table 6.9).

Table 6.9 **Causes of hyperkalaemia**		
Increased intake	**Decreased renal output**	**Movement of potassium out of cells**
Rapid blood transfusion Inappropriate intravenous replacement therapy Some dietary products contain high amounts of potassium, including chocolate and certain fruit (e.g. bananas)	Renal failure Addison's (adrenocortical insufficiency) Drugs: • ACE inhibitors • Potassium sparing diuretics • Ciclosporin	Muscle breakdown or disruption e.g. rhabdomyolysis, crush syndromes, trauma or malignant hyperthermia Acidosis Suxamethonium (will cause a rise of approximately 0.5 mmol/L, but this is exaggerated in patients with extra-junctional ACh receptors, such as burns patients or those with long-term immobility Familial periodic paralysis

Clinical features
• General symptoms such as muscle weakness and gastrointestinal upset.
• Myocardial depression and a spectrum of cardiac conduction problems, both atrial and ventricular.
• ECG changes such as peaked T waves, widened QRS complexes and slurring of ST segments into T waves.
• Plasma level >7 mmol/L may lead to ventricular dysrhythmias including ventricular fibrillation, and diastolic cardiac arrest.

Treatment
1. Potassium binding: using polystyrene sulphate resins PO or PR.
2. Intracellular movement of potassium:
   a. Using IV insulin to drive potassium into cells
   b. Sodium bicarbonate administration to exchange potassium for intracellular hydrogen ions
   c. Hyperventilation in artificially ventilated patients, by reducing serum hydrogen ion concentration and thus driving potassium into cells in exchange for intracellular hydrogen
   d. Nebulized or intravenous salbutamol, by increasing cellular uptake of potassium.
3. Physiological antagonism of potassium by intravenous calcium administration.
4. If severe or refractory, haemofiltration or dialysis may be required, especially in the setting of renal failure.

Limitations and complications
• Serum potassium samples may read artefactually high if the sample is haemolyzed or if there is a severe leucocytosis.
• The ratio of intracellular to extracellular potassium concentration is of more clinical relevance than an isolated plasma level.

Test: Serum magnesium

Indications
1. Preoperative biochemistry profile.
2. Renal failure.
3. Cardiac dysrhythmias.
4. Critical illness.
5. During therapeutic magnesium replacement therapy, e.g. for pregnancy-induced hypertension.

How it is done
Spectophotometric assay of serum sample.

Interpretation
Physiological principles
- Magnesium is a predominantly intracellular cation: 50% bone; 20% skeletal muscle; 29% heart, liver and other major organs; 1% extracellular fluid.
- It is a natural calcium antagonist; regulates intracellular potassium and calcium concentrations.
- Involved in enzymatic reactions in ATP synthesis and hydrolysis.
- Required for the synthesis of proteins and nucleic acids.
- Intravenous magnesium sulphate is used as an anti-arrhythmic, and as a vasodilator in pregnancy-induced hypertension and in the perioperative management of phaeochromocytoma.

Normal range
0.7–1.1 mmol/L.

Abnormalities and management principles
Hypomagnesaemia
Hypomagnesaemia is often found in association with hypocalcaemia and hypokalaemia (Table 6.10). It may be asymptomatic, but may present with the following clinical features:
- General: weakness and anorexia
- Cardiovascular: dysrhythmias (especially ventricular), prolonged QT interval, flattened T waves, short ST interval (occasionally)

Table 6.10 **Causes of hypomagnesaemia**	
Cause	Examples
Gastrointestinal loss	Diarrhoea and vomiting; malabsorption syndromes; malnutrition; small bowel disorders; chronic alcoholism
	Acute pancreatitis (magnesium sumps form in areas of fatty necrosis)
Renal loss	Loop and thiazide diuretics; acute alcohol intake; diabetic ketoacidosis; hypercalcaemia
Loop of Henle disorders	Acute tubular necrosis; renal transplantation; post-obstructive diuresis
Nephrotoxicity	Amphotericin B; aminoglycosides; ciclosporin A; cisplatin; pentamidine; digoxin
Other	SIADH; hyperaldosteronism

- Neurological: ataxia, tremor, carpopedal spasm, hyper-reflexia, hallucinations, convulsions.

Treatment

Identify cause and replace with oral or IV supplementation.

Hypermagnesaemia

True hypermagnesaemia is rare. It is usually due to renal insufficiency or exogenous ingestion (Table 6.11).

Table 6.11 **Causes of hypermagnesaemia**	
Cause	Examples
Renal	Renal failure of any aetiology
Exogenous administration	Purgatives (e.g. magnesium sulphate) Antacids (e.g. magnesium trisilicate) Therapeutic magnesium infusions/enemas
Drugs	Lithium Theophylline toxicity
Other	Adrenal insufficiency

Clinical features of hypermagnesaemia may occur at levels greater than 3–4 mmol/L and include:
1. Neurological: lethargy, drowsiness, areflexia, paralysis
2. Cardiovascular: hypotension, heart block, cardiac arrest.

Treatment with intravenous calcium may temporarily reverse toxic effects.

Limitations and complications

Serum levels are a poor reflection of total body magnesium as it is a predominantly intracellular ion.

Test: Serum calcium

Indications

1. Patients on calcium, phosphate or vitamin D therapy.
2. Renal failure.
3. Known abnormality of bone or magnesium homeostasis.
4. Pancreatitis.
5. Thyroid or parathyroid disease.
6. Critical illness (sepsis/immobility).
7. Patients on lithium or thiazides.
8. Coagulopathy.
9. Massive blood transfusion.

How it is done

- A number of studies have found free (ionized) calcium measurement to be a more clinically useful measurement of metabolic calcium disturbances than the commonly used total serum calcium measurement, which needs to be adjusted for serum albumin levels.
- Free (ionized) calcium can be measured either in the laboratory or in a blood gas analyzer using an ion-sensitive electrode technique.

Interpretation

Physiological principles

- Calcium is involved in coagulation, neuromuscular conduction, skeletal mineralization and the integrity of the cell membrane and transmembrane transport.
- 99% of the body's store of calcium is contained within bone and these stores buffer changes in serum calcium. Serum calcium content is divided equally between:
  - Bound calcium (i.e. bound to proteins and other ions)
  - Free ionized calcium.
- Calcium homeostasis is inextricably linked with that of phosphate and vitamin D and regulated by parathyroid hormone and calcitonin.

Normal range

1. Bound calcium (2.12–2.65 mmol/L; adjusted according to plasma protein levels – corrected by adding 0.02 mmol/L calcium for each g/L albumin below 40 g/L or by subtracting the same value for each g/L above albumin level 40 g/L.
2. Ionized calcium (0.8–1.1 mmol/L).

Abnormalities and management principles

Hypercalcaemia

Hypercalcaemia is due to either hyperparathyroidism or malignancy in over 90% of cases (Table 6.12).

Table 6.12 **Causes of hypercalcaemia**

Increased calcium absorption	Increased bony release	Miscellaneous
Increased dietary/exogenous intake of calcium Increased dietary/exogenous intake of vitamin D	Primary hyperparathyroidism Tertiary hyperparathyroidism Malignancy Hyperthyroidism	Immobility Sarcoidosis Addison's disease Phaeochromocytoma Drugs:Thiazide diuretics, lithium, theophylline toxicity

Clinical features

- Muscle weakness, malaise/depression, lethargy, confusion.
- Nephrolithiasis, nephrogenic DI, distal Renal Tubular Acidosis (RTA), renal failure.
- Peptic ulceration (due to excessive gastrin secretion), pancreatitis, constipation.
- Short QT syndrome; diabetes insipidus.

Management principles

1. Identifying and treating the cause.
2. Rehydration therapy (3–4 L crystalloid solution per day minimum) and loop diuretics.
3. Intravenous bisphosphonate therapy.

Treatment is usually mandatory for total serum corrected calcium levels above 3 mmol/L.

Hypocalcaemia

Commonest causes:

- Renal failure (due to increased serum phosphate levels)
- Hypoparathyroidism
- Vitamin D deficiency.

Other causes are listed in Table 6.13.

Table 6.13 Hypocalcaemia		
Decreased calcium absorption	Hyperphosphataemia (causing reduced ionized calcium levels)	Miscellaneous
Hypoparathyroidism Vitamin D deficiency Sepsis Hypomagnesaemia Fluoride poisoning	Renal failure Exogenous phosphate administration Rhabdomyolysis Tumour lysis syndrome	Pancreatitis EDTA infusion Hungry bone syndrome Acute respiratory alkalosis

Clinical features
- Neuromuscular problems (predominant clinical features):
  - Generalized myopathy
  - Extrapyramidal signs
  - Confusion and psychiatric symptoms
  - Tetany, seizures.
- Other:
  - Long QT syndrome
  - Papilloedema, cataracts.

Management
1. Identification and treatment of the underlying cause.
2. PO or IV replacement dependent on clinical situation.
3. Vitamin D supplementation in hypoparathyroidism, vitamin D deficiency or renal failure.

Limitations and complications
- Laboratory serum calcium levels may be misinterpreted with hypo- or hyperproteinaemia.
- Ionized calcium levels, as measured on arterial blood gas machines, will increase with acidosis and decrease with alkalosis. Thus, the use of a tourniquet for venous sampling or the presence of heparin, as in a blood gas syringe, may both cause an artefactual acidaemia and so an inaccurate ionized calcium result.

Test: Serum phosphate

Indications
1. Known disorder of phosphate metabolism.
2. Renal failure.
3. Patients on parenteral feeding.
4. Re-feeding syndrome.
5. Acid-base disturbance.
6. Malabsorption syndromes.
7. Rhabdomyolysis.

How it is done
Spectophotometric assay of serum sample.

Interpretation
Physiological principles
- Predominantly intracellular ion; forms part of the structure of cell membranes and plays essential roles in acid-base buffering, oxygen transport systems, energy storage and enzyme regulation.

- Regulated by renal excretion.
- Reduced phosphate excretion occurs in response to reduced intake, growth and thyroid hormones.

Normal range
Inorganic serum phosphate: 0.8–1.4 mmol/L.

Abnormalities and management principles

Hyperphosphataemia
Causes
The commonest cause of hyperphosphataemia is renal failure. Others are listed in Table 6.14.

Table 6.14 **Hyperphosphataemia**	
Acute phosphate loading	**Increased tubular re-absorption of phosphate**
Exogenous phosphate intake	Hypoparathyroidism
Rhabdomyolyis	Thyrotoxicosis
Lactic acidosis	Acromegaly
Ketoacidosis	Bisphosphonate treatment

Treatment
- Acute hyperphosphataemia:
  - Intravenous crystalloid rehydration
  - If severe, acetazolamide will increase phosphate excretion.
- Chronic hyperphosphataemia resulting from renal failure:
  - Phosphate binders such as calcium carbonate; low-phosphate diet
  - If severe, renal replacement therapy (dialysis or filtration).

Hypophosphataemia
Causes
Causes are listed in Table 6.15.

Table 6.15 **Causes of hypophosphataemia**		
Reduced intake/ intestinal absorption	**Increased renal excretion**	**Internal redistribution**
Reduced dietary intake, e.g. alcoholism	Primary hyperparathyroidism	Acute respiratory alkalosis
Total parenteral nutrition	Secondary hyperparathyroidism (nonrenal)	Hyperinsulinaemia
Magnesium or aluminium-containing antacids	Osmotic and thiazide diuretics	
Chronic diarrhoea or steatorrhoea	Acute plasma expansion	
Re-feeding syndrome	Vitamin D deficiency	

Clinical features
- Asymptomatic unless <0.6 mmol/L; may be associated with confusion, heart failure and even coma at extremely low levels.
- Muscle weakness, particularly of the respiratory muscles; may impair ventilatory weaning on the ICU.
- If the serum concentration <0.3 mmol/L, a reactive rhabdomyolysis may occur.

Test: Serum chloride

Indications
1. Metabolic acidosis.
2. Patients on intravenous fluid replacement therapy.
3. Patients on total parenteral nutrition.
4. Severe vomiting.

How it is done
Chloride ion-sensitive electrode (uses the same reference electrode as that used for pH measurement).

Interpretation
Physiological principles
- The body's predominant extracellular anion.
- Maintains electroneutrality, mainly as a counter to sodium; serum chloride generally increases and decreases with serum sodium.

Normal range
96–106 mmol/L.

Abnormalities and management principles
Hyperchloraemia
- Hyperchloraemia accompanying metabolic acidosis may occur with excessive infusion of normal saline and renal tubular acidosis.
- Other causes include hyperparathyroidism and hypernatraemia of any aetiology, including gastrointestinal upsets such as diarrhoea, dehydration, ileal loops and loss of pancreatic secretion.
- Drug causes include acetazolamide, ammonium chloride and triamterine.

Hypochloraemia
- Overhydration.
- Congestive cardiac failure.
- Syndrome of inappropriate secretion of ADH.
- Vomiting.
- Chronic respiratory acidosis or metabolic alkalosis of any aetiology.
- Addison's disease.
- Burns.
- Some instances of diuretic therapy.

Management principles
Identification and management of the underlying cause.

Test: Serum lactate

Indications
1. Metabolic acidosis.
2. Suspected or proven hypoperfusion (either generalized or specifically to the liver and/or intestinal tract).

How it is done
- Laboratory analysis using a venous or arterial blood sample.
- Lactate is oxidized by L-lactate peroxidase, producing hydrogen peroxide.
- This is then passed to a platinum electrode, which oxidizes the hydrogen peroxide, producing a current, the size of which is proportional to the lactate concentration.

Interpretation

Physiological principles
- Lactate is a by-product of anaerobic metabolism of pyruvate.
- Lactate levels may also rise as a result of reduced gluconeogenesis. Lactate is metabolized by the liver to bicarbonate, so a failure of this metabolism may also cause a rise in serum lactate.
- If a rise in serum lactate is also accompanied by a metabolic acidosis this is termed lactic acidosis.

Normal range
0.6–1.8 mmol/L.

Abnormalities

The causes of lactic acidosis are classified as either Type A (associated with tissue hypoxia) or Type B (without tissue hypoxia) (Table 6.16).

Table 6.16 **Causes of lactic acidosis**	
Type A (tissue hypoxia)	**Type B (no tissue hypoxia)**
Hypoxaemia	Hepatic failure
Anaemia	Renal failure
Hypoperfusion of any origin (e.g. haemorrhage, sepsis, hypovolaemia)	Diabetes mellitus
Cardiac failure	Drug-induced: e.g. salicylate overdose, biguanides, alcohols
Ischaemic bowel	Total parenteral nutrition
	Inborn errors of metabolism
	Glycogen storage disorders

Management principles
- Management of lactic acidosis predominantly involves identification and treatment of the underlying cause.
- Initial supportive management includes optimization of tissue oxygen delivery with adequate oxygenation, cardiac output and haemoglobin concentration.

Test: Serum bicarbonate

Indications
Any suspected acid-base disturbance.

How it is done
Calculated from the plasma pH and PCO_2, as measured by the pH and Severinghaus electrodes in a blood gas analyzer.

Interpretation

Physiological principles
- Bicarbonate is an anion that is a major component of the body's predominant buffer system.
- It is formed from the dissociation of carbonic acid as a part of a three-stage chemical reaction, which is catalyzed by carbonic anhydrase.
- Bicarbonate is completely filtered in the glomerulus and then reabsorbed, predominantly in the proximal tubule, via the formation of carbonic acid; the degree of this reabsorption is determined by total body acid-base balance.

Normal range
24–33 mmol/L.

Abnormalities and management principles
See Chapter 2.

Limitations and complications
See Chapter 2.

Investigation of salt and water disturbance

Test: Serum osmolality

Indications
1. Renal impairment.
2. Serum sodium derangement.
3. Suspicion of diabetes insipidus or SIADH.

How it is done
1. Estimation using the formula:
   Plasma osmolality = [Glucose] + [urea] + 2 × [sodium]
   (mosmol/kg)   (mmol/L)   (mmol/L)   (mmol/L)
2. Laboratory determination of depression of freezing point.
3. Laboratory measurement of osmotic pressure.
4. Laboratory determination of serum ionic concentrations using flame photometry.

Data presented as
Numerical data: units mosmol/kg solvent.

In the case of plasma, the solvent is water.

Interpretation
Physiological principles
- Osmolality – the number of osmoles per kilogram solvent.
- Osmolarity – the number of osmoles per litre of solution

where osmole refers to the molecular weight of a substance divided by the number of freely moving particles in solution.
- In the plasma, the presence of proteins and fats mean that the values for osmolarity and osmolality are slightly different.
- In health, plasma osmolality is maintained within a narrow range by a number of homeostatic mechanisms involving osmoreceptors, which respond to changes by the stimulation of antidiuretic hormone.

Normal range
280–305 mosmol/kg.

Abnormalities and management principles
Syndrome of inappropriate ADH secretion (SIADH)
This is characterized by low plasma osmolality and sodium, high urine sodium and urine/plasma osmolality ratio >1.

It may be caused by:
- Ectopic vasopressin secretion (from malignancies, including lymphoma or carcinoma of bronchus, pancreas, colon, prostate)
- Pulmonary disease (e.g. tuberculosis, pneumonia)
- Neurological disorders (e.g. meningitis, encephalitis, tumour, head injury, neurosurgery)
- Drugs (e.g. chlorpropamide, oxytocin, carbemazepine, certain antidepressants).

Treatment
- Identify and treat underlying cause.
- Water restrict; demeclocycline may be used to block the renal effects of ADH.

Diabetes insipidus (DI)
This causes a high serum osmolality and presents with polyuria and polydipsia associated with reduced ADH activity.

This may be due to:
- Cranial DI: hyposecretion of ADH – e.g. due to head injury, brain tumours, neurosurgery or, rarely, familial cranial DI
- Nephrogenic DI: renal unresponsiveness to the effects of ADH – e.g. related to drugs such as lithium, demeclocycline and gentamicin. Patients are unable to concentrate their urine in response to water deprivation.

Treatment
Depends on the cause.
- Cranial DI is treated with desmopressin, a synthetic ADH analogue.
- Nephrogenic DI is treated with thiazide diuretics.

Limitations and complications
- Pathologically high levels of alcohols, proteins, triglycerides and mannitol will make the calculation of osmolality using the above formula inaccurate, as these molecules are not accounted for.
- Urine osmolality should also be measured to confirm diagnosis of SIADH or DI.

Assessment of thyroid function

Test: Serum thyroid hormones measurement

Indications
Investigation of thyroid function.

How it is done
Serological immunoassay of thyroxine, thyronine and thyroid-stimulating hormone.

Interpretation
Physiological principles
- Thyroxine (L-thyroxine, T4) is an amine hormone produced by the thyroid gland under the influence of thyroid-stimulating hormone (TSH), which is produced in the pituitary. T4 has a half life of 7 days.
- Thyroxine is enzymatically cleaved to T3 (L-thyronine) in the thyroid gland and in the circulation; T3 is the active form and has a half life of one day.

Normal ranges
- Serum thyroxine (T4) = 4.6–12 μg/dL.
- Free thyroxine (T4) = 0.7–1.9 ng/dL.

- Serum T3 = 80–180 ng/dL.
- Free T3 = 230–619 pg/dL.
- Serum TSH = 0.5–6 μmol/mL.

Abnormalities and management principles

Hyperthyroidism

Causes

The commonest causes are characterized by an overactive gland and thus normal or increased radio-iodine uptake; these are Graves' disease, toxic (hot) nodule and toxic multinodular goitre administration. Drugs that can induce hyperthyroidism include amiodarone and oestrogens.

Clinical features are listed in Table 6.17.

Table 6.17 **Clinical features of hyperthyroidism**	
Cardiovascular	Dyspnoea; atrial fibrillation; high-output cardiac failure
Musculoskeletal	Proximal myopathy, periodic paralysis; osteoporosis; hypercalcaemia
Blood	Leucopenia; microcytic anaemia

It is characterized by an increase in serum T4 measurements; TSH may or may not be suppressed depending on the cause.

- Medical management is with carbimazole or propyluracil, which prevent formation of thyroid hormones.
- Iodine therapy temporarily inhibits hormone release and is often given for 2 weeks before thyroidectomy.
- Beta adrenoceptor antagonists have dual effect, by reducing the conversion of thyroxine to the active tri-iodothyronine, and also by counteracting the systemic effects of hyperthyroidism.
- Surgical removal of the thyroid gland requires adequate preoperative medical control of hyperthyroidism, in order to prevent precipitation of a thyroid crisis.

Hypothyroidism

Causes

- Total or partial thyroidectomy.
- Drugs – e.g. amiodarone, aspirin, phenytoin, interferon, frusemide, lithium.
- Autoimmune diseases are 10 times more common in females, and the incidence increases with age.
- It is characterized by a reduction in T4/T3 levels, and will be accompanied by a high TSH if the hypothyroidism is due to intrinsic thyroid disease or drugs affecting the thyroid.
- It may rarely be caused by pituitary disease, in which case the TSH will also be low.

Clinical features are listed in Table 6.18.

- Hypothyroidism may present as a medical emergency in the form of a myxoedema coma.
- It is treated with oral thyroxine replacement or, in the emergency setting, with intravenous T3.

Assessment of glycaemic control

Test: Serum glucose

Indications

1. Diabetes mellitus.
2. Any acute or critical illness, in particular, sepsis, acute pancreatitis.

Table 6.18 **Clinical features of hypothyroidism**	
General	Serous effusions (ascites, pleural, pericardial or joint effusions); hypothermia
Cardiovascular	Hypercholestrolaemia and ischaemic heart disease; bradycardia; cardiomegaly ECG changes include low-voltage complexes and T wave flattening/inversion
Respiratory	Hypoventilation
Musculoskeletal	Muscular chest pain; muscular cramps; raised creatinine kinase
Blood	Macrocytic anaemia; microcytic anaemia in context of menorrhagia in women

3. Reduced level of consciousness.
4. Glycogen storage diseases.

How it is done

Laboratory assay

Several methods exist. In one such method D-glucose is oxidized in the presence of glucose oxidase, producing hydrogen peroxide and glucono-δ-lactone. Hydrogen peroxide is then passed to a platinum electrode, where it is oxidized; the magnitude of the resultant current is proportional to the glucose concentration.

Glucose reagent sticks

The same oxidation reaction is employed, producing hydrogen peroxide. In the case of reagent sticks, the hydrogen peroxide then oxidizes a dye, which produces a colour change that can be compared against a chart.

Interpretation

Physiological principles

In health, blood sugar is maintained within a narrow range by various neuroendocrine response systems including the sympathetic nervous system, insulin and glucagon.

Normal range

Fasting blood glucose: 4.1–7 mmol/L.

Abnormalities and management principles

Hyperglycaemia

Hyperglycaemia is defined as fasting plasma glucose greater than 7.0 mmol/L. Causes are listed in Table 6.19.

Chronic hyperglycaemia

- Diabetes mellitus causes multisystem problems, and is a leading cause of morbidity and mortality in the Western world.
- Diabetes may be classified as:
  - Type 1: due to failure of insulin secretion; most commonly diagnosed in childhood or adolescence
  - Type 2: due to insulin resistance and is usually associated with defective insulin secretion

Table 6.19 Causes of hyperglycaemia

Causes	Examples
Pancreatic insufficiency	Diabetes mellitus (types 1 and 2) Acute or chronic pancreatitis or pancreatectomy Sepsis Cystic fibrosis
Neuroendocrine response causing increased circulating catecholamines, growth hormone, glucocorticoids, glucagon	Trauma, burns, critical illness Stress response to surgery
Insulin resistance	Type 2 diabetes mellitus Polycystic ovary syndrome Acromegaly, Cushing's syndrome or glucagonomas Phaeochromocytoma
Exogenous administration of glucose	Total parenteral nutrition (TPN), enteral nutrition
Drugs	Steroids, thiazide diuretics, octreotide

- Type 3: encompasses all other specific forms of diabetes, including those related to genetic beta cell defects, genetically related insulin resistance, pancreatic disease, hormones or drugs.
- Type 4: gestational diabetes

Acute hyperglycaemia
- Diabetic ketoacidosis is frequently precipitated by a concomitant illness.
- Hyperosmolar nonketotic coma is a more common presentation of hyperglycaemia in elderly patients. Progressive dehydration due to polyuria results in a very high plasma osmolality accompanying severe hyperglycaemia, but with little or no ketonuria.
- Management of both conditions involves slow correction of fluid, glycaemic and electrolyte abnormalities.

Acute hypoglycaemia
- Hypoglycaemia in diabetic patients may occur in those treated with either insulin or oral sulphonylureas.
- Hypoglycaemia in nondiabetic patients is rare, but can occur in association with hepatic disease, alcohol, hypoadrenalism and certain tumours (e.g. insulinomas, IGF-2 secreting tumours).
- Postprandial hypoglycaemia is well documented in patients post gastrectomy.

Tight glycaemic control
- Evidence from several major studies has found there to be outcome benefit, both in terms of morbidity and mortality from controlling blood glucose in surgical critically ill patients.
- There is still some debate over whether 'tight' glycaemic control is more beneficial than 'moderate' glycaemic control; however, most studies use a target blood glucose range of 4–8 mmol/L.

Limitations and complications
1. Glucose reagent sticks tend to be less accurate at lower glucose levels.
2. Falsely high glucose results may occur due to contamination of the testing sample, for example, with glucose-containing contaminants on the skin from where a blood sample is obtained.

Test: Glycosylated haemoglobin (HbA1C)

Indications

Monitoring of long-term glycaemic control.

Data presented as

A percentage of glycosylated haemoglobin relative to red cell haemoglobin.

Interpretation

Physiological principles
- Red cell haemoglobin is nonenzymatically glycated at a rate that relates to overall level of glucose.
- It has been found to correlate well with the risk of microvascular complications and so is a valuable tool in the assessment of long-term glycaemic control.

Normal range
There is no standardized assay of HbA1C and interpretation should be made in conjunction with local guidelines.

Abnormalities and management principles

- The commonest cause of a high HbA1C is poor glycaemic control secondary to diabetes mellitus of any aetiology.
- However, abnormalities in HbA1C may occasionally be due to some haemoglobinopathies and disorders of red cell metabolism.

Investigation of the hypothalamic–pituitary axis

Test: Short synacthen test

Indications

Suspected adrenocortical insufficiency:
1. Sepsis/critical illness
2. Addison's disease
3. Long-term steroid usage
4. Pituitary disease or surgery.

How it is done

1. Baseline serum sample for cortisol assay.
2. Intravenous administration of 250 μg synthetic adrenocorticotrophin (ACTH) – tetracosactrin.
3. Serum cortisol assay at 30 minutes following ACTH administration.

Serum cortisol samples are laboratory analyzed by radioimmunoassay.

Data presented as

Numerical value for cortisol assay; units nmol/L.

Interpretation

Physiological principles
The administered dose of tetracosactrin should maximally stimulate the adrenal cortex. In the case of adrenal insufficiency, the adrenal cortex is unable to respond to this stimulus, resulting in a subnormal rise in serum cortisol levels.

Normal range

Post-ACTH administration cortisol level >500 nmol/L.

Abnormalities

The causes of adrenocortical insufficiency may be divided into:

1. Primary adrenal failure (Addison's disease). This may have a variety of aetiologies including autoimmune (most common), infiltration from TB, malignancy or amyloidosis, critical illness, haemorrhage or infarction. Autoimmune Addison's may be associated with other autoimmune disorders.
2. Secondary adrenal failure. Most commonly due to either abrupt withdrawal of long-term steroid therapy, ACTH deficiency due to pituitary disease or surgery.

Adrenal insufficiency as demonstrated by an inadequate increment in serum cortisol in response to a short synacthen test may result in a variety of clinical, biochemical and haematological abnormalities. The clinical features differ in acute and chronic adrenocortical insufficiency (Table 6.20).

Table 6.20 **Acute versus chronic adrenocortical insufficiency**

Acute	Chronic
Clinical features • Abdominal and muscular pain • Hypotension • Psychosis	Clinical features • Malaise and muscle weakness • Weight loss • Diarrhoea and vomiting • Postural hypotension • Increased susceptibility to infection
Haematological features • Eosinophilia • Lymphocytosis • Normocytic anaemia	
Biochemical features • Raised serum urea • Hyponatraemia • Hypoglycaemia • Hyperkalaemia • Hypercalcaemia • Hypochloraemia	

Management principles

• Severe acute adrenocortical insufficiency may present with circulatory collapse.
• Longer term management involves steroid replacement therapy, initially with intravenous hydrocortisone, and then subsequently with oral prednisolone if required.

Measurement of hormones: Phaeochromocytoma

Test: Plasma and urine catecholamines and their metabolites

Indications

Known or suspected phaeochromocytoma.

How it is done

1. Plasma assays

Laboratory assay of venous blood sample for plasma epinephrine and norepinephrine levels.

2. Urine assays

Laboratory assay of 24-hour urine sample for urinary epinephrine, norepinephrine and dopamine levels. Their urinary metabolites, vanillylmandelic acid (VMA), metanephrine and normetanephrine, may also be measured.

Interpretation

Physiological principles

- Phaeochromocytomas are rare tumours of the sympathetic nervous system that are found in either the adrenal medulla or on sympathetic ganglia.
- They may secrete one or a combination of epinephrine, norepinephrine and dopamine; extraadrenal tumours do not secrete epinephrine.
- Symptoms include headache, sweating, palpitations, psychosis. Other symptoms or signs of hypertension, and sometimes hypotension, including postural hypotension, especially if the tumour secretes epinephrine.
- Patients may also present with signs or symptoms of glucose intolerance and cardiomyopathy.

Management principles

Resection of phaeochromocytomas involves careful anaesthetic preparation.

1. Complete preoperative alpha-blockade using phentolamine or phenoxybenzamine.
2. Subsequently, complete beta-blockade.
3. Prevention of intraoperative hypertension using vasodilators such as GTN, sodium nitroprusside or magnesium sulphate, and intraoperative tachy-arrhythmias using beta-blockers or amiodarone.
4. Goal-directed fluid resuscitation, particularly after tumour resection.
5. Postoperative high-dependency unit (HDU)/intensive care unit (ICU) admission.

Limitations

- Plasma catecholamine levels may be normal or only slightly elevated in up to a third of patients with phaeochromocytoma.
- Slight elevations of urinary and serum catecholamines and their metabolites may occur in a number of patients with poorly controlled systemic hypertension that is not due to phaeochromocytoma.
- False-positive urinary VMA results may occur because of concurrent therapy with methyldopa, levodopa or labetolol. It may also occur in patients with clonidine withdrawal, hypoglycaemia, raised intracranial pressure and after strenuous exercise.
- Various medications may cause false-positive results in urinary and serum catecholamine and metanephrine levels.

A variety of physiological stresses and pathophysiological processes may also cause false-positive urinary catecholamine and plasma catecholamine and metanephrine levels including the stress response to surgery, myocardial infarction, critical illness and depression.

Further investigations

- Clonidine suppression testing (i.e. the measurement of plasma free normetanephrine before and after administration of clonidine) may aid in the diagnosis.
- Preoperative tumour localization is carried out using CT scanning, radioactive meta-iodobenzyl guanidine (MIBG) scintigraphy and/or selective venous catheterization.

Measurement of hormones: Carcinoid tumours

Test: Urinary 5-hydroxyindole acetic acid (5-HIAA)

Indications
Known or suspected carcinoid tumour or carcinoid syndrome.

How it is done
Laboratory assay of 24-hour urine samples using high-performance liquid chromatography with electrochemical detection.

Interpretation
Physiological principles
- Carcinoid tumours are common, being an incidental finding in 1% of post-mortems. 85% of carcinoid tumours are found in the terminal ileum; they are rarely found outside the GI tract, in the lungs and gonads.
- Carcinoid tumours secrete serotonin and kinins but remain asymptomatic until hepatic metastases are present, resulting in carcinoid syndrome, which is a rare diagnosis. The presence of hepatic metastases impair serotonin metabolism, resulting in a variety of symptoms and signs, including flushing in association with wheezing, sweating, vasodilatation and resultant hypotension. They may also cause episodic diarrhoea and commonly lead to weight loss.
- Right-sided cardiac failure may result from endocardial fibrosis of the tricuspid and pulmonary valves (left-sided cardiac failure may occur in the presence of bronchial carcinoid or an Atrial Septal Defect (ASD)).

Normal range
3–15 mg/day. There is a correlation between tumour mass and 5-HIAA production.

Management principles
Anaesthetic management of carcinoid resection
- Cardiostable induction and maintenance with invasive arterial and central venous pressure monitoring.
- Consider cardiac output monitoring using oesophageal Doppler or similar.
- Intraoperative management revolves around the prevention of hypo- or hypertension, and bronchospasm.
- Postoperative ICU/HDU management.

Limitations
- Bananas, kiwi fruit, pineapples and a variety of nuts, all of which are serotonin rich, may cause false-positive results.
- Certain drugs, including salicylates, paracetamol and L-dopa may also affect the assay.

Further investigations
- Preoperative tumour localization is carried out using CT, MRI or PET scanning.
- Echocardiography is recommended if there are signs of cardiac involvement.

Investigation of allergic reactions

Test: Serum mast cell tryptase measurement

Indications
Suspected anaphylactic or anaphylactoid reaction.

How it is done
Enzyme immunoassay.

Interpretation
Physiological principles
Tryptase is a neutral protease that is found almost exclusively in mast cells. It exists in two structural forms (α and β); β–tryptase is normally involved in airway homeostasis, vascular contraction and relaxation, gastrointestinal motility and smooth muscle activity and in coagulation. Unlike histamine, tryptase remains elevated in the plasma for some hours after an anaphylactic reaction.

Normal range
<11.4 ng/mL.

Abnormalities and management principles
- Anaphylaxis (a type I immune reaction) and anaphylactoid reactions (involving complement released as well as mast cell degranulation) both lead to the release of histamine, serotonin, kinins and leukotrienes amongst other vasoactive substances.
- An important clinical difference between the two types of reaction is that anaphylaxis requires prior exposure and thus sensitization to the culprit agent, whereas anaphylactoid reactions do not.
- The management of suspected anaphylactic and anaphylactoid reactions is outlined in guidelines published by the Association of Anaesthetists of Great Britain and Ireland (AAGBI).

Limitations and complications
- At least three serial mast cell tryptase samples are required to be able to diagnose anaphylaxis, looking for an initial high value followed by serial decay.
- Mast cell tryptase assay does not distinguish between anaphylactic and anaphylactoid reactions.

Test: Serum and urine histamine assay

Indications
Suspected anaphylactic or anaphylactoid reaction.

How it is done
Enzyme immunoassay of either a 2-mL blood sample (non-EDTA bottle), 5 mL urine sample or 24-hour urine collection.

Data presented as
Numerical value. Units: ng/mL for random urine and blood sample; µg/24 hours for 24-hour urine collection.

Interpretation
Physiological principles
Histamine is a low-molecular-weight molecule produced by the decarboxylation of histidine. It is actively released from mast cells and basophils as part of anaphylactic and anaphylactoid reactions, but is also found throughout many body tissues and organs. Peak levels occur within 10 to 20 minutes of exposure, and then rapid decay to baseline occurs within 60–90 minutes. Thereafter, histamine may be detected in the urine.

Normal range
- Whole blood: 20–200 ng/mL.
- Random urine: 0–88 ng/mL.
- 24-hour urine: 0–118 µg/24 hours.

Abnormalities and management principles

See under mast cell tryptase.

Limitations and complications

Histamine assay does not differentiate between anaphylactic and anaphylactoid reactions.

TOPIC ⑦

Haematology and coagulation

Topic Contents

Common first tests 130
  Test: Full blood count and peripheral
    blood smear (PBS) **130**
  Test: Group and screen/crossmatch **135**
Laboratory tests of coagulation 137
  Tests: Prothrombin time (PT)/
    international normalized ratio (INR),
    activated partial thromboplastin time
    (APTT) and thrombin time (TT) **137**
  Test: Fibrinogen **139**
  Test: D-dimers and fibrin degradation
    products **140**
  Test: Anti-Xa assay **141**
  Test: Factor inhibitor assay/mixing
    studies **141**
  Test: Hypercoagulation screen **141**
Point-of-care tests of coagulation 142
  Test: Activated clotting time (ACT) **142**

  Test: High-dose thrombin time (HiTT) **142**
Haemoglobinopathies 143
  Test: Sickledex **143**
  Test: Haemoglobin electrophoresis/
    high-performance liquid chromatography
    (HPLC) **144**
**Viscoelastic measurement of
  haemostasis 144**
  Test: Thromboelastography/
    thromboelastometry **144**
Laboratory platelet function monitors 150
  Test: Optical light transmission platelet
    aggregometry (LTA) **150**
**Point-of-care platelet function
  monitors 151**
  Test: PFA-100 **151**

Common first tests

Test: Full blood count and peripheral blood smear (PBS)

Indications

- To show abnormalities in the production, life span, and destruction of blood cells and aid in the diagnosis of anaemia, polycythaemia, thrombocytosis, thrombocytopenia, leucopaenia and leucocytosis.
- To help diagnose infection.
- As a preoperative baseline in cases with expected significant blood loss (see NICE guidelines at http://www.nice.org.uk).
- As a guide to blood/platelet transfusion.

How it is done

- Blood is taken into an EDTA tube and analyzed, ideally within 4 hours.
- Automated blood counters using either forward angle light scatter or impedance analysis to provide:
  - Enumeration of erythrocytes, leucocytes (5 part differential count) and platelets
  - Quantification of haemoglobin (Hb) by spectrophotometry in lyzed sample
  - Erythrocyte mean cell volume (MCV), haematocrit (Hct), red cell distribution width (RDW), a measure of cell size scatter
  - Derived parameters include mean cell haemoglobin (MCH) and mean corpuscular haemoglobin concentration (MCHC).
- The counter flags samples that need further analysis with a PBS and a manual count or examination of morphology.

Interpretation

Normal adult ranges.

See Table 7.1.

Table 7.1 **Normal adult ranges for blood values**

	Male	Female*
Haemoglobin (g/dL)	13–18.0	11.5–16.5
RBCs ($\times 10^{12}$/L)	4.5–6.5	4.0–5.8
Hct (%)	0.40–0.52	0.37–0.47
MCV (fL)	84–96	84–96
MCH (pg)	27.0–32.0	
MCHC (g/dL)	27.0–32.0	
Platelets ($\times 10^9$/L)	150–400	
WBCs ($\times 10^9$/L)	4.0–11.0	
Neutrophils ($\times 10^9$/L)	2.0–7.5	
Lymphocytes ($\times 10^9$/L)	1.5–4.0	
Monocytes ($\times 10^9$/L)	0.2–0.8	
Eosinophils ($\times 10^9$/L)	0.04–0.4	
Basophils ($\times 10^9$/L)	0.0–0.1	
Reticulocytes (% or 10^9/L)	0.5–2.5 or 20–80	

*In pregnancy the Hb may fall as low as 9 g/dL in the third trimester. RBCs, red blood cells; Hct, haematocrit; MCV, mean cell volume; MCH, mean cell haemoglobin; MCHC, mean corpuscular haemoglobin concentration; WBC, white blood cell.

Abnormalities

Anaemia: Low haemoglobin
See Table 7.2.

Polycythaemia: Increased haemoglobin/haematocrit
See Table 7.3.

Table 7.2 The anaemias

Type of anaemia	Differential diagnosis	Peripheral blood smear (PBS)	Comment
Microcytic MCV <80 fL	Iron deficiency anaemia	Anisocytosis, Poikilocytosis, Elliptocytosis	Hypochromic (low MCH) Low serum ferritin, low iron and raised total iron binding capacity (TIBC)
	Thalassaemia	Polychromasia, target cells, basophilic stippling	
	Anaemia of chronic disease		Due to chronic inflammatory and infective conditions
Normocytic MCV 80–100 fL	Bleeding	Polychromasia	
	Haemolysis; may be: • Hereditary or acquired • Immune or non-immune • Extravascular or intravascular	Polychromasia, spherocytes, schistocytes, bite cells	Low haptoglobin Raised LDH, bilirubin and reticulocytes
	Anaemia of chronic disease		Especially associated with renal failure
Macrocytic megaloblastic MCV >100 fL	Vitamin B12/folate deficiency	Oval macrocytes, Howell-Jolly bodies, basophilic stippling	Serum B12 low Raised LDH Pernicious anaemia: intrinsic factor antibodies Reduced red cell folate (reflects total body folate status)
Macrocytic normoblastic MCV >100 fL	Liver disease and excessive alcohol consumption		
	Hypothyroidism		
	Drug induced		e.g. hydroxyurea
	Myelodysplastic syndrome	Ringed sideroblasts (iron stain), nuclear abnormalities of leucocytes	
	Marked reticulocytosis		e.g. in haemolysis

Table 7.3 Polycythaemia

True polycythaemia	Secondary polycythaemia	Apparent or spurious polycythaemia
Polycythaemia rubra vera, (PRV)	Inappropriate erythropoietin secretion in benign & malignant renal disorders and by some tumours	Secondary to cigarette smoking, obesity, excess alcohol or hypertension

Thrombocytopenia: Platelet count $<150 \times 10^9$/L
See Table 7.4.

Table 7.4 Causes of thrombocytopenia

Failure of production	Increased consumption	Pseudothrombocytopenia
Drugs & chemicals Viral infection, e.g. HIV Radiation Aplastic anaemia Leukaemia Marrow infiltration Megaloblastic anaemia Liver disease	Idiopathic thrombocytopenic purpura (ITP) Disseminated intravascular coagulation (DIC) Infection Haemorrhage & transfusion Systemic lupus Some leukaemias & lymphoma Heparin Hypersplenism Thrombotic thrombocytopenic purpura (TTP) Haemolytic uraemic syndrome	Caused by clumping: can be excluded by examination of PBS and citrate sample (clumping due to EDTA)

Thrombocytosis: Platelet count $>450 \times 10^9$/L
See Table 7.5.

Table 7.5 Causes of thrombocytosis

Primary myeloproliferative disorder	Secondary reactive disorder
Essential thrombocythaemia PRV Idiopathic myelofibrosis	Haemorrhage Acute & chronic infection Inflammatory disease Post splenectomy Trauma/surgery Iron deficiency anaemia Malignancy

Leucopenia: WBC $<4.0 \times 10^9$/L
- It is uncommon for absolute leucopenia to be due to an isolated deficiency of any cell other than the neutrophil.
- The risk of infection is closely related to the absolute neutrophil count.

- *Neutropenia* – neutrophils $<2.0 \times 10^9$/L.
- *Lymphopenia* – lymphocytes $<1.5 \times 10^9$/L.

See Table 7.6.

Table 7.6 Leucopenias

Neutropenia		Lymphopenia
Congenital causes	**Acquired causes**	
Benign chronic neutropenia (Yemenite Jews & people of African descent) Rare – Kostmann's syndrome, cyclic neutropenia	Drugs – cytotoxic agents, anticonvulsants, thyroid inhibitors, antibiotics, clozapine, procainamide, hydroxychloroquine, penicillamine, NSAIDs Post-infectious – usually after viral infection: • Severe sepsis • Autoimmune • Felty's syndrome (rheumatoid arthritis) • Splenomegaly	Acute infections Cardiac failure Tuberculosis Uraemia Lymphoma, carcinoma Systemic lupus erythematosus Corticosteroids HIV

Leucocytosis

Detection of a leucocytosis by the automated counter needs confirmation with a PBS and manual count. See Table 7.7.

Table 7.7 Causes of leucocytosis

Neutrophilia ($>7.5 \times 10^9$/L)	Lymphocytosis ($>4.0 \times 10^9$/L)	Eosinophilia	Basophilia
Infection/ inflammation Drugs – corticosteroids, epinephrine Myocardial infarction Exercise Stress including after surgery Cigarette smoking 'Leukaemoid reaction': response to severe infection	Viral infection Infectious mononucleosis CMV, hepatitis A Chronic infection with TB, brucellosis, secondary syphilis CLL, ALL, occasionally NHL	Drugs Parasite infections Asthma and allergic reactions Vasculitides Metastatic cancer Hypereosinophilic syndrome	Myeloproliferative disorders Inflammatory disorders Drugs Viral infection Hypothyroidism

ALL, acute lymphoblastic leukaemia; CLL, chronic lymphocytic leukaemia; NHL, non-Hodgkin lymphoma.

Management principles

- The full blood count is often performed unnecessarily as a preoperative screening tool. Various studies have shown that this is a waste of resources although some would argue that it is indicated in all premenopausal women because of the higher incidence of anaemia.
- NICE guidelines are available indicating those patients who should have a full blood count performed, mainly those with significant comorbidity or undergoing major surgery.
- Abnormal results may need manual verification or a PBS to provide further information.

Limitations and complications

- 5% of the population lie outside the 'normal' reference range.
- People of Afro-Caribbean descent display significantly lower haemoglobin, WBC, neutrophil and platelet count.
- Individuals may show substantial change from their baseline without falling outside 'normal range'.

Test: Group and screen/crossmatch

Indications

- To determine a patient's ABO blood group, and to screen serum for the presence of antibodies to common red cell antigens.
- To allow provision of appropriate red cell concentrate (RCC) and blood products in order to avoid transfusion reactions.

How it is done

- 'Group' – determines which ABO and Rh antigens are present on patient's red blood cells (RBCs). RBCs are incubated with commercially available antibodies (anti-A, anti-B), which react with antigens if present and cause agglutination. The patient's serum is then incubated with A and B cells to determine the presence of anti-A and anti-B antibodies. (See Table 7.8)

Table 7.8 **ABO blood group antigens present on RBC and IgM antibodies present in serum**

	Group A	Group B	Group AB	Group O
Antigens present	A antigen	B antigen	AB antigen	No antigens
Antibodies present	Anti-B	Anti-A	No antibodies	Anti-A & Anti-B
UK incidence	42%	8%	3%	47%

- 'Screen' – utilizes the indirect Coomb's test (indirect antiglobulin test). Serum is incubated with a wide range of RBCs that together exhibit a comprehensive range of surface antigens. If antibodies are present they will cause agglutination.
- Crossmatch – may be electronic or serological. An electronic crossmatch is used in uncomplicated cases with a negative antibody screen. A serological crossmatch requires RBCs from the donor unit to be incubated with the patient's serum, which will cause agglutination if the unit is not compatible.

Interpretation

Data presented as
- A, B or O blood group and Rhesus (Rh) status, e.g. O+, AB−.

Physiological principles
- Blood type is determined by the presence or absence of inherited antigenic material on the surface of RBCs; the ABO blood group system and Rh blood group system are the two most likely to cause harmful immunologically mediated reactions if noncompatible blood is transfused.
- ABO system. The A and B antigens are produced from a common precursor, the H antigen. Either, both or none may be present. Anti-A or anti-B IgM antibodies are produced in the first years of life possibly by sensitization to environmental substances such as food, viruses and bacteria.
- Rhesus system. The most significant Rh antigen is the Rh D antigen, which is either present (Rh D positive, RhD+) or not (Rh D negative, RhD−). IgG and IgM anti-D antibodies are formed in RhD-negative individuals through a sensitizing event.

Management principles

- ABO compatibility. When considering blood group compatibility for transfusion it is the recipient **antibodies** and **donor** antigens that are important. For example, group AB individuals have A and B antigens on the surface of their RBCs; their blood serum does not contain any antibodies against either A or B antigen so they can receive blood from any group (in theory, AB being preferable). Blood group O individuals have neither antigen but both anti-A and anti-B antibodies therefore will cause agglutination of the donor RBCs if they are given anything other than group O blood (Table 7.9).

Table 7.9 **Red blood cell compatibility**								
Recipient blood type	Donor RBC must be:							
AB+	O−	O+	A−	A+	B−	B+	AB−	AB+
AB−	O−		A−		B−		AB−	
A+	O−	O+	A−	A+				
A−	O−		A−					
B+	O−	O+			B−	B+		
B−	O−				B−			
O+	O−	O+						
O−	O−							

- Rhesus compatibility. An RhD-negative patient with no antibodies could only receive RhD-positive blood once, as this would lead to the formation of antibodies and potentially hazardous transfusion reactions if they were to receive it again. If an RhD-negative woman develops antibodies and becomes pregnant with an RhD-positive child, these antibodies can cross the placenta and cause haemolytic disease of the newborn. Therefore rhesus-positive blood or platelets should never be given to RhD-negative women of childbearing age or patients with rhesus D antibodies. Platelets can be given with anti-D cover in emergencies.
- Plasma compatibility. Donor-recipient compatibility is the opposite of blood compatibility. Type O plasma (fresh frozen plasma, FFP) can only be given to type O recipients; Type AB can be given to individuals of any blood group (Table 7.10).

Table 7.10 **Plasma compatibility**	
Recipient blood type	Donor plasma must be:
AB	AB
A	A or AB
B	B or AB
O	O, A, B or AB

- There are usually local policies in place for the routine ordering of preoperative G&S or crossmatched blood that take into account the planned surgery, estimated blood loss and need for transfusion.
- Guidelines are available for the transfusion of blood and blood products published by The Association of Anaesthetists of Great Britain and Ireland (AAGBI) and British Committee for Standards in Haematology (BCSH) and advice should be sought from a haematologist where necessary.

Laboratory tests of coagulation

Tests: Prothrombin time (PT)/international normalized ratio (INR), activated partial thromboplastin time (APTT) and thrombin time (TT)

Indications
- Part of coagulation screen often ordered preoperatively.
- Assessment of synthetic liver function.
- Assessment of coagulopathy in disseminated intravascular coagulation (DIC) and massive blood transfusions.
- INR used to monitor warfarin therapy.
- APTT used to monitor unfractionated heparin therapy.
- TT used in diagnosis of hypo/dysfibrinogenaemia.

How it is done
- Platelet poor plasma (PPP) obtained from citrated blood sample (9:1 ratio).
- PT/INR – thromboplastin and calcium added to PPP and time to fibrin formation measured by a photo-optical or electromechanical device; this equals the prothrombin time (PT). To standardize results the PT is compared to a reference value, which gives the INR.
- APTT – PPP, phospholipid and calcium are added to kaolin and the time to fibrin formation measured.
- TT – thrombin added to plasma and clotting time measured in seconds.

Interpretation
Normal range/graph
- PT = 10–14 seconds.
- INR = 0.9–1.2.
- APTT = 25–35 seconds.
- TT = <15 seconds.

Physiological principles
- Coagulation was traditionally thought to consist of 'intrinsic' and 'extrinsic' pathways with a final common pathway. This has now been replaced with the cell-based model of haemostasis which comprises three stages of initiation, amplification and propagation.
- At the site of vascular injury tissue factor (TF) expressed on extravascular cells forms a TF/VIIa complex that activates factors X to Xa and IX to IXa.
- Factor Xa converts factor V to Va and forms a Xa/Va complex on the TF cell, which converts prothrombin to thrombin (initiation).
- Thrombin activates platelets and factors VIII, V and XI.
- Factor VIII circulates in combination with von Willebrand factor (vWF) which acts as a carrier molecule to transport factor VIII to the platelet surface.
- Activated platelets bind cofactors VIIIa and Va with their respective enzymes IXa and Xa to form a prothrombinase complex, which causes a thrombin burst to take place on the surface of the activated platelet (amplification).
- Thrombin converts fibrinogen to fibrin and the haemostatic plug comprised of platelets and fibrin strands is formed (propagation and stabilization).
- Control mechanisms exist to limit fibrin formation to the site of injury including TF pathway inhibitor, the protein C and S system and antithrombin III.
- Disturbances in these mechanisms can lead to thrombotic disorders.

Abnormalities
See Table 7.11.

Table 7.11 **Coagulation abnormalities**		
Prolonged INR	**Prolonged APTT**	**Prolonged TT**
Due to deficiency of factor I, II, V, VII or X: • Warfarin anticoagulation therapy • Vitamin K deficiency resulting in deficiency of vitamin K dependent factors II, VII, IX and X • Liver disease • Coagulopathy secondary to DIC* • Coagulopathy secondary to massive blood transfusion • Dilutional coagulopathy • High-dose unfractionated heparin therapy • Fibrinogen deficiency • Haemorrhagic diseases of the newborn	Due to deficiency of Factor VIII, IX, XI or XII: • Unfractionated heparin therapy • Haemophilia A, B or C (factor VIII, IX or XI deficiency, respectively) • Lupus anticoagulant (actually prothrombotic but binds to phospholipid in test sample) • Coagulopathy secondary to DIC • Coagulopathy secondary to massive blood transfusion • Von Willebrand disease	Prolonged due to thrombin inhibition: • Heparin • Fibrin degradation products (FDP) • Lupus anticoagulant

Disseminated intravascular coagulopathy: DIC may complicate massive tissue injury, sepsis and some pregnancy-related complications. The normal anticoagulant and fibrinolytic systems are overwhelmed resulting in disseminated microvascular thrombi with consumption of platelets and coagulation factors leading to a haemorrhagic state. The fibrinolytic system is activated to dissolve the fibrin thrombi, resulting in the formation of D-dimers and fibrin degradation products (FDP), which have a further anticoagulant action.

Management principles
- Preoperatively.
- Determine cause for prolonged INR.
- Stop warfarin and start heparin if anticoagulation essential.
- Current guidelines for the emergency reversal of Warfarin therapy include vitamin K and prothrombin complex concentrates (PCC) containing plasma-derived factors II, VII, IX and X.
- In the presence of bleeding or to correct the INR prior to surgery/invasive procedures treatment options include:
  - FFP to maintain INR 1.5–1.8 unless there is evidence of microvascular ooze
  - PCC.
- Protamine for heparin overdosage.

Further investigations
- Liver function tests.
- Full blood count (FBC) (monitor platelet count on heparin).
- Fibrinogen level to exclude hypofibrinogenaemia.
- Mixing studies to check for possible factor deficiencies or inhibitors.
- Specific factor deficiencies.
- Lupus/anticardiolipin antibodies.
- Fibrin degradation products (FDPs).

Limitations and complications
- Underfilling sample tube alters the anticoagulant:blood ratio of 9:1.
- High or low haematocrit alters the APTT.
- Heparin contamination prolongs PT and APTT.
- Haemolysis, lipaemia, hyperbilirubinaemia and hyperproteinaemia produce errors in the optical endpoint analysis.
- APTT is not suitable for high-dose heparin, e.g. on cardiopulmonary bypass.

Test: Fibrinogen

Indications
- Diagnosis of acquired/hereditary fibrinogen deficiencies.

How it is done
- Most automated analyzers produce a *derived* fibrinogen level from PT, APTT and TT.
- *Clauss* method uses a high concentration of thrombin, which is added to dilute patient plasma, converting fibrinogen into a fibrin clot. The amount of fibrinogen in the sample is inversely proportional to the clotting time.

Interpretation
Normal range
1.5–4.0 g/L.

Abnormalities
See Table 7.12.
- <1.0 g/L may be associated with bleeding.

Table 7.12 **Abnormalities of fibrinogen**	
Elevated fibrinogen	Fibrinogen deficiencies
Pregnancy Acute phase reactions	Congenital Acquired: • Advanced liver disease • DIC due to excessive thrombin generation • Thrombolytic therapy • Massive blood transfusion

Management principles
- In a bleeding patient if fibrinogen level <1.0 g/L give cryoprecipitate, which contains 350 mg of fibrinogen, factor VIII, von Willebrand factor, factor XIII and fibronectin or fibrinogen concentrate.
- With massive transfusion fibrinogen levels fall rapidly and cryoprecipitate should always be given as well as FFP.

Further investigations
- Usually done in conjunction with a coagulation screen.
- FDPs.
- D-dimers.

Test: D-dimers and fibrin degradation products

Indications
- Diagnosis of DIC.
- Diagnosis of deep vein thrombosis/pulmonary embolism (DVT/PE).

How it is done
- Latex agglutination assay.
- Enzyme-linked immunosorbent (ELISA) assay.

Interpretation
Normal range/graph
- D-dimers <0.5 μg/mL.
- FDP <5 μg/mL.

Physiological principles
- Fibrinolysis is mediated by plasmin, which degrades fibrin clots into D-dimers and FDPs.

Abnormalities
Elevated D-dimers/FDP:
- Massive tissue injury, sepsis
- Malignancy
- Intrauterine death
- DVT/PE.

Management principles
- DIC – identify cause, support coagulation with blood, FFP, cryoprecipitate and platelets as necessary.
- Antithrombin concentrates or recombinant activated protein C have also been used.

- Heparin has been used in the treatment of DIC but is controversial.
- DVT/PE – anticoagulation.

Further investigations
- Coagulation screen.
- Fibrinogen.

Limitations and complications
- Not specific.
- Latex agglutination tests are not sensitive to exclude DVT/PE.
- Moderate increases of D dimers in major surgery do not necessarily indicate a pathological state.
- Rheumatoid factor may cause false positives.

Test: Anti-Xa assay
Indications
- Monitoring low-molecular-weight heparin (LMWH).
- Monitoring unfractionated heparin when APTT cannot be used, e.g. if lupus anticoagulant present.
- Different from factor X activity assay, which tests for rare factor X deficiency.

Interpretation
Normal range
- Unfractionated heparin: therapeutic 0.3–0.7 anti-Xa units/mL; prophylactic 0.1–0.4 anti-Xa units/mL.
- LMWH: therapeutic 0.5–1.0 anti-Xa units/mL; prophylactic 0.2–0.4 anti-Xa units/mL.

Test: Factor inhibitor assay/mixing studies
Indications
- To identify specific factor deficiencies or the presence of inhibitors.

How it is done
- Patient's serum mixed with normal serum and APTT measured.
- A 50:50 mix will correct a factor deficiency.
- A 50:50 mix will not correct the APTT in the presence of an inhibitor.

Test: Hypercoagulation screen
Indications
- Diagnosis of acquired or congenital hypercoagulable conditions leading to venous or arterial thromboses.

How it is done
- Panel of tests including:
  - Protein C & S levels
  - Activated protein C resistance & factor V Leiden mutation
  - Antiphospholipid antibody
  - Homocysteine.

Management principles
- Patients at risk of venous or arterial thromboembolism may require anticoagulation.

Point-of-care tests of coagulation

Test: Activated clotting time (ACT)

Indications
- Monitor high doses of unfractionated heparin used in cardiopulmonary bypass (CPB), interventional radiology, haemofiltration and critical care.
- Assess adequacy of heparin reversal by protamine.

How it is done
- Sample of whole blood added to a glass tube containing an activator and a small magnet and slowly rotated at 37° in the analyzer.
- As the blood clots the magnet is pulled away from a detection switch and this signals the ACT.
- Other devices use a cuvette, which only needs two drops of blood.

Interpretation
Normal range/graph
- Normal ACT = 107 ± 13 seconds.
- Prolonged ACT:
  - Heparin
  - Hypothermia
  - Haemodilution
  - Excess protamine administration.

Management principles
- Adjust dose of heparin to achieve an ACT of at least 4 times baseline (normally >480 seconds).

Limitations and complications
- ACT is relatively insensitive to low doses of heparin.
- High ACT values of >600 do not have a linear relationship with heparin dose.
- Affected by hypothermia/haemodilution.
- As protamine may affect the ACT, a prolonged ACT after the appropriate dose of protamine should not generally be treated.
- Aprotinin prolongs celite-activated ACT so ACT should be kept >750 seconds; kaolin-activated ACT is unaffected by aprotinin.

Test: High-dose thrombin time (HiTT)

Indications
- Monitor high doses of unfractionated heparin used in cardiopulmonary bypass (CPB), interventional radiology, haemofiltration and critical care.

How it is done
- Assay contains high levels of thrombin to cleave fibrinogen directly and produce a fibrin clot independently of other plasma coagulation factors.
- Thrombin is inhibited by heparin therefore the HiTT is prolonged in presence of heparin.

Limitations and complications
- Hypo/dysfibrinogenaemia prolongs HiTT.
- Limited shelf life of thrombin reagent.

Haemoglobinopathies

Test: Sickledex

Indications
- Screening test for sickle cell anaemia/sickle cell trait (see NICE guidelines).

How it is done
- Blood is mixed with sodium metabisulphite, a reducing agent that induces sickling in susceptible cells. These can be viewed under a microscope within 20 minutes.

Interpretation

Data presented as
- Positive or negative test.

Physiological principles
- This is an autosomal recessive condition in which the beta chain of haemoglobin A has valine substituted for glutamine at position 6 (HbS).
- At low oxygen tensions deoxygenated HbS aggregates producing abnormal, rigid 'sickle'-shaped cells, which can impede blood flow.
- Sickled cells adhere to the vascular endothelium resulting in chronic endothelial inflammation and damage.
- Sickle cells haemolyze resulting in anaemia.

Abnormalities
A positive test indicates presence of HbS but does not differentiate between:
- Sickle cell trait – heterozygous condition HbS/HbA
- Sickle cell anaemia – homozygous HbS/HbS
- Other haemoglobinopathy in which patients are heterozygous for HbS and another abnormal Hb, e g HbSC.

Management principles
- All patients of African and Afro-Caribbean descent should have screening by Sickledex test prior to anaesthesia if sickle status unknown.
- Eastern Mediterranean, Middle Eastern and Asian people should also be considered.
- Preoperative advice from haematologists with regards to the need for 'top up' or exchange transfusion in patients with sickle cell disease. The hazards of exchange transfusion may outweigh the benefits unless the patient is considered high risk for developing a crisis and complications. Preoperative transfusion aims for a haematocrit of 30% and HbS less than 30%.
- Sickling can be induced by hypoxia, acidosis, dehydration, hypothermia and presence of desaturated HbS therefore perioperative management includes keeping patients warm and well-hydrated, administering supplemental oxygen and maintaining an adequate cardiac output.
- The use of tourniquets is controversial and most authorities advise against their use unless absolutely necessary.
- Antibiotic prophylaxis is important as risk of infection is higher.

Further investigations
- FBC and PBS to look for anaemia (normocytic) and characteristic morphological changes.
- Haemoglobin electrophoresis.
- U&E, urinalysis, liver function tests and chest x-ray to investigate signs of end organ damage.

Limitations and complications
- Indicates presence of HbS not the diagnosis of Sickle cell disease.
- Is positive if HbS is more than 20% of total haemoglobin, so has limited use if recently heavily transfused or <1 year old.

Test: Haemoglobin electrophoresis/high-performance liquid chromatography (HPLC)

Indications
- Diagnosis of haemoglobinopathy.

How it is done
- Haemoglobin electrophoresis is performed at an alkaline pH. At this pH, haemoglobin, a negatively charged protein, will migrate to the anode.
- Normal and abnormal haemoglobins separate from each other on the basis of charge and produce distinct bands that also allow quantification.

Interpretation
Data presented as
- Type and percentage of haemoglobins present.

Abnormalities
- Sickle cell disease – HbS present (see Sickledex test).
- Thalassaemia – genetic disorder resulting in abnormal rates of production of alpha and beta haemoglobin chains. The gene/promoter deletions result in a spectrum of clinical conditions ranging from asymptomatic to death in utero.

Management principles
- As above for sickle cell anaemia/trait.
- Obtain haematology advice.
- There are some case reports of difficult intubation associated with thalassaemia due to ectopic marrow expansion in the bones of the face.

Further investigations
- FBC: Sickle cell anaemia, normocytic anaemia.
- Thalassaemias: hypochromic, microcytic anaemia with normal iron levels.
- Other tests may be required (e.g. echocardiogram to assess pulmonary hypertension) after discussion with a haematologist.

Viscoelastic measurement of haemostasis

Test: Thromboelastography/thromboelastometry

Indications
- Point-of-care test of global coagulation.
- Diagnosis of hypo- or hypercoagulability, platelet function and primary/secondary fibrinolysis.
- To guide blood product and antifibrinolytic drug administration.

How it is done
- Two main instruments perform similar assays:
  - Thromboelastography (TEG, Haemoscope Corp, IL, USA; Fig. 7.1) results in a thromboelastograph trace

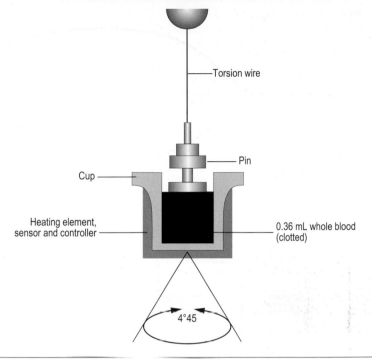

Fig. 7.1 TEG cup attached to pin and torsion wire.

- Thromboelastometry (ROTEM, Pentapharm, Milton Keynes, UK) results in a thromboelastogram trace.
- A small quantity of blood is placed in a heated cup.
- A pin is suspended within the cup connected to a detector system, a torsion wire in the TEG system and an optical detector in the ROTEM system.
- The cup and pin are oscillated relative to each other.
- Initially when no clot exists the motion of the cup does not affect the pin and the resulting trace is a straight line. As fibrin forms characteristic traces are obtained.
- Modifications:
  - Addition of 'activators', e.g. kaolin, celite or tissue factor, which allow more rapid results
  - Heparinase-coated cups to evaluate the effects of exogenous or endogenous heparins
  - Functional fibrinogen tests.

Interpretation

Data presented as
- Graphical trace (Fig. 7.2) and descriptive data. See Table 7.13.

Normal range
- Normal range differs depending on instrument and whether activators are used.

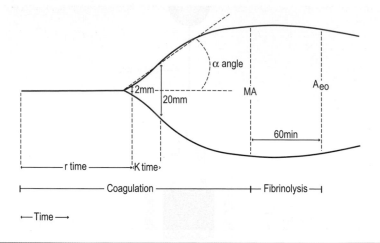

Fig. 7.2 TEG trace showing common parameters.

Table 7.13 **Nomenclature used for TEG and ROTEM**

	TEG	ROTEM
Measurement period		RT
Clot time-latency time from placing blood in cup until clot starts to form (2 mm amplitude)	Reaction time r	Clotting time (CT)
Period from 2 mm to 20 mm Amplitude	K	Clot formation time (CFT)
Alpha angle	α	α
Maximum angle		Clot formation rate (CFR)
Maximum strength	Maximum amplitude (MA)	Maximum clot firmness (MCF)
Time to maximum strength	TMA	MCF-t
Amplitude at set time	A30, A60	A5, A10...
Clot elasticity	G	Maximum clot elasticity (MCE)
Maximum lysis		Maximum lysis (ML)
Lysis at fixed time	LY30, LY60	CL30, CL60

Physiological principles

• The cell-based model of haemostasis involves the exposure of tissue factor (TF) and formation of a TF/factor VIIa complex, which causes activation of other factors and the ultimate conversion of prothrombin to thrombin.

- Thrombin activates platelets and further thrombin activation takes place on the platelet surface.
- Control mechanisms exist to limit fibrin formation to the site of injury; disturbances in these mechanisms can lead to thrombotic disorders.

Normal

See Fig. 7.3.

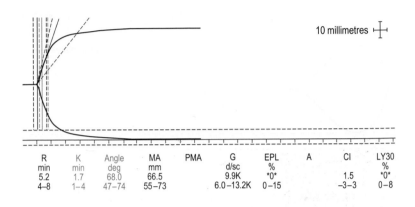

R min	K min	Angle deg	MA mm	PMA	G d/sc	EPL %	A	CI	LY30 %
5.2	1.7	68.0	66.5		9.9K	*0*		1.5	*0*
4–8	1–4	47–74	55–73		6.0–13.2K	0–15		–3–3	0–8

Fig. 7.3 Normal TEG trace.

Abnormalities

Hypocoagulable
See Fig. 7.4.

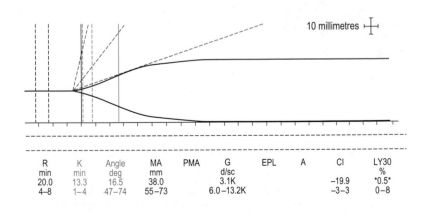

R min	K min	Angle deg	MA mm	PMA	G d/sc	EPL	A	CI	LY30 %
20.0	13.3	16.5	38.0		3.1K			–19.9	*0.5*
4–8	1–4	47–74	55–73		6.0–13.2K			–3–3	0–8

Fig. 7.4 Hypocoagulable TEG trace.

- R, K = prolonged.
- α, MA = decreased.
- Factor deficiency.
- Anticoagulant therapy.
- Thrombocytopenia.

Primary(hyper) fibrinolysis
See Fig. 7.5.

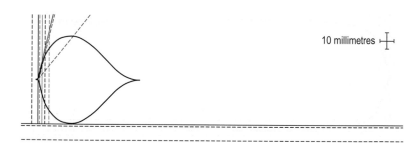

10 millimetres ⊢⊢

Fig. 7.5 Primary fibrinolysis.

- R = normal.
- MA = continuous decrease.
- LY60 >15%.
- e.g. trauma, advanced liver disease.

Secondary fibrinolysis
See Fig. 7.6.

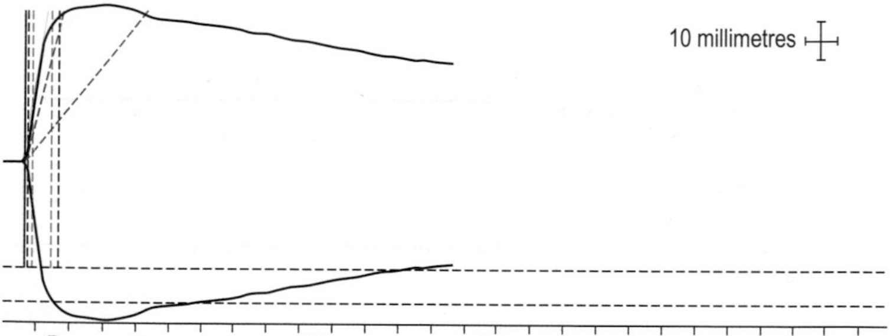

10 millimetres ⊢⊢

R min	K min	Angle deg	MA mm	PMA	G d/sc	EPL %	A	CI	LY30 %
3.4	1.0	79.0	82.5		23.6K	12.5		5.7	12.5
4–8	1–4	47–74	55–73		6.0–13.2K	0–15		–3–3	0–8

Fig. 7.6 Secondary fibrinolysis.

- Hypercoagulable state with secondary fibrinolysis.
- LY60 >15%.
- e.g. DIC.

Hypercoagulable
See Fig. 7.7.

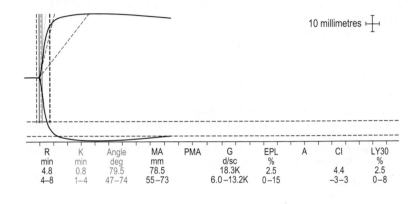

10 millimetres ⊢⊣

R min 4.8 4-8	K min 0.8 1-4	Angle deg 79.5 47-74	MA mm 78.5 55-73	PMA	G d/sc 18.3K 6.0-13.2K	EPL % 2.5 0-15	A	CI 4.4 -3-3	LY30 % 2.5 0-8

Fig. 7.7 Hypercoagulable TEG trace.

- R, K = decreased.
- MA, α = increased.

Management principles
- Treatment algorithms based on thromboelastograph/thromboelastogram results have been shown to reduce blood and blood product administration in cardiac surgery, liver transplantation and critical care.
- In general:
  - Prolonged R – give FFP 10–15 mL/kg
  - Prolonged R, heparinase trace normal – give protamine
  - Reduced MA – give desmopressin (e.g. DDAVP), platelet transfusion
  - Primary fibrinolysis – give antifibrinolytic drugs, e.g. tranexamic acid, aprotinin
  - Secondary fibrinolysis – determine cause and treat appropriately
  - Low α angle/low fibrinogen – give cryoprecipitate.
- Hypercoagulable traces may be used to identify patients at risk of peri-/postoperative thrombotic events.

Further investigations
- FBC/Hb if patient bleeding.
- Thrombotic screen may be indicated with hypercoagulable trace.

Limitations and complications
- Native samples need to be analyzed within 4 minutes of venepuncture.
- Citrated samples should be analyzed between 1 and 4 hours so are not always appropriate for point of care testing when immediate results are needed.

- Citrated samples do not always show good correlation with native samples.
- High interuser variability, therefore tests should be performed in as standardized a way as possible and interpreted in the clinical setting.

Laboratory platelet function monitors

Test: Optical light transmission platelet aggregometry (LTA)

Indications
- 'Gold standard' for assessment of platelet function.
- Diagnosis of congenital and acquired platelet disorders.

How it is done
- Anticoagulated blood is used to prevent thrombin-mediated activation of platelets and fibrinogen cleavage.
- Blood is centrifuged to obtain platelet rich plasma.
- Different platelet agonists are added to stimulate platelet aggregation; ADP, arachidonic acid, collagen, ristocetin.
- Changes in light transmittance after platelet stimulation are measured to give the degree of platelet aggregation and compared to platelet poor plasma.

Interpretation
Data presented as
- Percentage aggregation.

Physiological principles
- Platelets are involved in normal haemostasis and the haemostatic plug.
- They adhere to exposed endothelial surfaces at the site of a vascular injury and become activated.
- Thrombin generation takes place on the platelet surface and converts fibrinogen to fibrin
- Activated platelets undergo conformational change of GPIIb/IIIa receptors, which bind fibrin to form the platelet/fibrin haemostatic plug.

Abnormalities
See Table 7.14.

Table 7.14 **Platelet abnormalities**		
Congenital platelet dysfunction	**Acquired platelet dysfunction**	**Antiplatelet drugs**
Failure of production or function(rare)	Renal failure Liver failure Post cardiopulmonary bypass Myeloproliferative disorders	Cyclo-oxygenase inhibitors (e.g. aspirin) GPIIb/IIIa inhibitors (e.g. abciximab) Thienopyridines (e.g. clopidogrel, ticlopidine) Phosphodiesterase inhibitors (e.g. cilostazol)

Management principles
- Stop antiplatelet drugs if indicated before a surgical procedure.
- Platelet transfusion is needed if the patient is actively bleeding and has poor platelet function.

- DDAVP has been used when poor platelet function occurs in the context of renal failure or von Willebrand disease.

Further investigations
- Specialist haematological referral if appropriate.

Limitations and complications
- Laboratory based; long sample preparation time.
- Artificial activation of platelets during centrifugation.
- Interference from lipaemia.
- Does not take account of other cellular components of blood.

Point-of-care platelet function monitors

Test: PFA-100
Various point-of-care platelet function monitors are available. The PFA-100 is described in detail.

Indications
- Assessment of adequacy of antiplatelet therapy.
- Assessment of platelet function prior to invasive/surgical procedure.
- Guide to platelet transfusion in bleeding patients.

How it is done
- The PFA-100 simulates a vascular injury and measures the time taken for a platelet plug to occlude an aperture in a membrane that is impregnated with collagen and either epinephrine (EPI) or adenosine diphosphate (ADP). This is the closure time C-EPI CT or C-ADP CT.

See Fig. 7.8.

Interpretation
Data presented as
See Table 7.15.

Physiological principles
- See LTA.

Abnormalities
See Table 7.16.

Management principles
- As above.

Further investigations
- Confirmation by platelet aggregometry if necessary.

Limitations and complications
- Results are not always consistent when compared to gold standard platelet aggregometry and may give false negatives with clopidogrel.
- Closure time linearly prolongs as platelet counts fall below 100×10^9.
- Not accurate if haematocrit low.

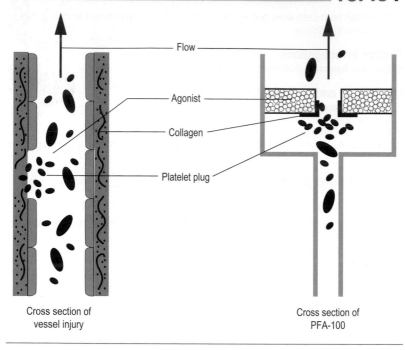

Cross section of
vessel injury

Cross section of
PFA-100

Fig. 7.8 Cross section of PFA-100 showing simulated vessel injury.

Table 7.15 PFA-100 **data.**		
Closure time		
Normal		**Nonclosure**
C-EPI CT 77–163 seconds		>300 seconds
C-ADP CT 64–114 seconds		

Table 7.16 **Causes of platelet abnormalities**	
Prolonged C-EPI CT	**Prolonged C-ADP CT**
Aspirin	Clopidogrel
	von Willebrand disease
	Renal failure

TOPIC 8

The labour ward

Topic Contents

Fetal well-being: Antenatal investigations 153
Test: Cardiotocograph (CTG) **153**
Test: Fetal scalp blood sampling **158**
Test: Fetal lactate **159**
Test: Fetal electrocardiogram (ECG) analysis **160**

Fetal well-being: Postnatal investigations 160
Test: Cord blood sampling **160**
Test: APGAR scoring **161**
Maternal well-being 162
Test: Electrocardiogram **162**
Test: Antenatal tests in the UK **162**
Test: Blood tests during pregnancy **163**

Fetal well-being: Antenatal investigations

The main aim of fetal monitoring is to identify the fetus at risk in order to allow sufficient time to intervene thereby preventing permanent injury or death from occurring. Currently the optimal method for assessing fetal well-being during labour and delivery has not been determined.

Test: Cardiotocograph (CTG)

Indications
For factors in high-risk pregnancies see Table 8.1.

How it is done
A cardiotocograph simultaneously records both the fetal heart rate (FHR) and uterine contractions.

External monitoring
The FHR is derived from a Doppler ultrasound transducer that detects fetal heart movements and a pressure transducer that records the frequency and duration (but not strength) of uterine contractions. Both transducers are applied externally to the maternal abdominal wall.

Internal monitoring
The FHR is monitored via an electrode that is inserted transcervically to penetrate the fetal scalp and the frequency, duration and strength of uterine contractions are recorded via a fine intrauterine pressure catheter. Internal monitoring requires cervical dilatation and rupture of the membranes. Internal FHR monitoring provides a more accurate measurement of beat to beat and baseline variability than external monitoring.

Table 8.1 **Factors involved in high-risk pregnancies**

Maternal factors	Fetal factors
Pre-eclampsia/hypertension	Fetal growth restriction
Diabetes	Prematurity
Other significant maternal medical conditions	Oligohydramnios
Maternal pyrexia	Abnormal Doppler artery velocimetry
Previous caesarean section	Multiple pregnancies
Post-term pregnancy (>42 weeks)	Meconium-stained liquor
Prolonged membrane rupture (>24 hours)	Breech presentation
Induced/augmented labour	
Antepartum haemorrhage	
Epidural analgesia	

A hybrid of internal measurement of fetal heart rate with external monitoring of contractions may be performed.

Data presented as
The CTG trace (Fig. 8.1) shows two lines:
- The upper line is a record of the fetal heart rate in beats per minute
- The lower line is a recording of uterine contractions

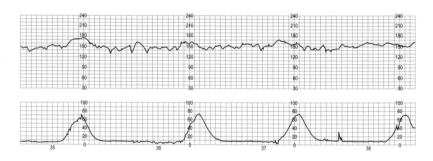

Fig. 8.1 Normal CTG.

Interpretation
Physiological principles
- An electronic method of determining fetal heart rate, presence and duration of uterine contractions in addition to the reaction of the fetus to contractions.
- Assessments are made of fetal heart rate, variability of heart rate, presence or absence of accelerations and decelerations.

The fetus requires an adequate supply of oxygen via the placenta and umbilical vein. Interruption of this blood supply may compromise a fetus without adequate reserve. Uterine contractions or cord compression may interrupt this blood supply. Fetal hypoxaemia may present itself as changes to the CTG tracing as discussed below.

Definitions

Baseline FHR

The average FHR, excluding accelerations and decelerations, determined over a 5–10-minute period. Normal valves are 110–160 beats per minute (bpm).

Bradycardia

A baseline heart rate of less than 110 bpm (Fig. 8.2). A profound and sustained decrease in FHR is indicative of fetal distress.

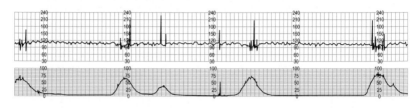

Fig. 8.2 CTG of fetal bradycardia.

Tachycardia

A suspicious tachycardia is defined as being between 160 and 180 bpm, whereas a pathological recording is above 180 bpm. Fetal tachycardias may be associated with fetal distress, maternal pyrexia and/or intrauterine infection.

Baseline variability

This is the minor fluctuation in baseline fetal heart rate. It is measured by estimating the difference in beats per minute between the highest peak and lowest trough of fluctuation in a 1-minute segment of the trace. The normal baseline variability is >5 bpm between contractions. Decreased or absent variability (Fig. 8.3) reflects decreased fetal central nervous system activity (associated with fetal sleep cycles or maternal drug administration, e.g. opioid, magnesium, benzodiazepines). However sustained reduction in variability may indicate fetal hypoxaemia/acidosis.

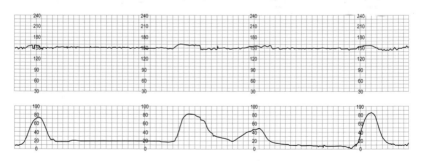

Fig. 8.3 CTG of loss of variability.

Accelerations

This is defined as a transient increase in heart rate >15 bpm for at least 15 seconds. Accelerations are normal indicating fetal responsiveness. Two accelerations in 20 minutes is considered a reactive trace. The absence of accelerations with an otherwise normal CTG is of uncertain significance.

Decelerations

These may either be normal or pathological:

- *Early decelerations* (Fig. 8.4A) occur at the same time as uterine contractions and are thought to result from fetal head compression, transient elevation of intracranial pressure and reflex increased vagal tone. They are considered benign.
- *Late decelerations* (Fig. 8.4B) start during the mid–end period of the contraction and end after the completion of the contraction. Their presence suggests fetal hypoxaemia/acidosis.

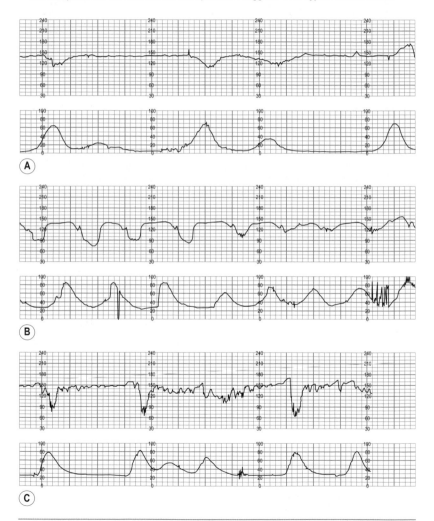

Fig. 8.4 CTGs of (A) early decelerations, (B) late decelerations and (C) variable decelerations.

- *Variable decelerations* (Fig. 8.4C) have a variable temporal relationship to uterine contractions or occur in isolation. They are thought to result from umbilical cord compression.

Normal values, abnormalities and management principles

See Table 8.2 and Table 8.3.

Table 8.2 **Categorization of fetal heart traces**	
Category	Definition
Normal	A CTG where all four features fall into the reassuring category
Suspicious	A CTG whose features fall into one of the nonreassuring categories and the remainder of the features are reassuring
Pathological	A CTG whose features fall into two or more nonreassuring categories or one or more abnormal categories

From Royal College of Obstetricians and Gynecologists (2001) The use of electronic fetal monitoring: the use and interpretation of cardiotocography in intrapartum fetal surveillance. http://www.rcog.org.uk

Table 8.3 **Categorization of fetal heart rate (FHR) features (Table 2.3 RCOG guidelines)**				
Feature	Baseline (bpm)	Variability (bpm)	Decelerations	Accelerations
Reassuring	110–160	≥5	None	Present
Nonreassuring	100–109 161–180	<5 for ≥40 but <90 minutes	Early deceleration Variable deceleration Single prolonged deceleration <3 minutes	Absent
Abnormal	<100 >180 Sinusoidal pattern ≥10 minutes	<5 for ≥90 minutes	Atypical variable decelerations Late decelerations Single prolonged deceleration >3 minutes	Absent

From Royal College of Obstetricians and Gynaecologists (2001) The use of electronic fetal monitoring: the use and interpretation of cardiotocography in intrapartum fetal surveillance. http://www.rcog.org.uk

Management principles

RCOG guidelines recommend:
- Those falling into the suspicious category should follow the conservative approach
- Conservative measures include:
  - Maternal supplemental oxygen
  - Maternal repositioning (thereby reducing aorto-caval compression or dislodgement of occult cord prolapse)

- Administration of intravenous fluid bolus (non-glucose crystalloid 500 mL) unless concern about possible intravascular fluid overload (e.g. pre-eclampsia)
- Stopping/reducing oxytocin augmentation as blood flow to the placenta is reduced during contractions
- Consideration of tocolysis (e.g. terbutaline 0.25 mg subcutaneously).
- Those patients in the pathological category should undergo further assessment with fetal blood sampling with a view to urgent delivery if necessary.
- However if fetal compromise is present, this should not delay immediate delivery, ideally within the accepted standard of 30 minutes.

Note that all CTG tracings should be kept as part of the birth record for a minimum of 25 years for medicolegal reasons.

Limitations and complications

- FHR monitoring is accurate at confirming a healthy non-acidotic fetus, however it is poor at predicting a hypoxaemic acidotic fetus. This is due to the low prevalence of asphyxia in labour and the fact that the positive predictive valve of any test is directly proportional to the prevalence of the disease it is predicting.
- Although continuous intrapartum FHR monitoring was introduced in order to reduce perinatal mortality and cerebral palsy, it has failed to achieve this aim. The likely explanation is that only 10% of cases of cerebral palsy are thought to have intrapartum causes. Its use, however, does appear to have reduced the incidence of neonatal seizures.
- There is considerable intra- and inter-observer variation in interpretation of the CTG even amongst experts, increasing likelihood of both false-positive and false-negative results.
- Maternal drugs affect FHR monitoring (e.g. beta-blockade and spinal opioids associated with fetal bradycardia).
- The mother is confined to bed (with application of monitor belts or fetal scalp electrode) unless telemetry available.
- The use of intrapartum CTG monitoring has been associated with an increase in interventional/operative delivery, without necessarily being justified.
- Early rupture of membranes may be required for internal monitoring via a fetal scalp electrode and this may cause fetal distress (the procedure can cause increased direct pressure of the fetal head on the cervix causing intense and prolonged contractions).
- Fetal scalp electrode application carries an infective risk.

Further investigations

- Fetal blood sampling.
- Fetal scalp lactate measurement.
- Fetal electrocardiogram analysis.

Test: Fetal scalp blood sampling

Indications

- Assessment of fetal acid-base balance and adequacy of oxygenation.
- Usually other markers of fetal hypoxia are present such as CTG abnormality.
- The evidence supports that with pathological fetal heart rate the use of fetal scalp blood sampling as an additional surveillance is associated with less vaginal operative deliveries, and improved short-term neonatal outcome.

How it is done
- Requires ruptured membranes, cervical dilatation >3 cm.
- Left lateral or occasionally lithotomy position.
- Small cut made in fetal scalp skin and 30–40 µL of blood collected.

Interpretation
Physiological principles
- Impaired fetal oxygen supply causes anaerobic metabolism of glucose.
- This in turn causes a metabolic acidaemia via pyruvate and lactate.

Abnormalities and management principles
- Normal scalp blood pH 7.25–7.35.
- Scalp pH >7.25 and fetal heart trace remains non-reassuring:
  - Continue to observe labour
  - Repeat scalp sampling every 2–3 hours.
- Scalp pH 7.21–7.24 and fetal heart trace remains non-reassuring:
  - Repeat scalp sample in 15–30 minutes or consider rapid delivery if rapid decrease in pH since last sample.
- Scalp pH <7.20:
  - Immediate delivery indicated.
- Assessment of fetal pH should be in context of clinical scenario.

Limitations and complications
- Breech presentations (debatable relationship between buttock and scalp pH).
- Avoid in parturient with HIV, hepatitis B, herpes simplex.
- Avoid in fetal bleeding disorders and prematurity (<34 weeks' gestation).
- Often contaminated causing rejection of sample (amniotic fluid, etc).
- Uncomfortable for patient.

Test: Fetal lactate
Indications
- Assessment of fetal well-being.
- Adjunct to CTG monitoring.

How it is done
- See fetal blood sampling above.
- Less blood needed – 5 µL versus 30–40 µL.
- Lower failure rate than fetal blood sampling.
- Hand-held devices available.

Interpretation
Physiological principles
- Lactate is produced as glucose is metabolized anaerobically in absence of oxygen.
- Good correlation between fetal pH and lactate levels.
- Lactate may be better at predicting poor outcomes than pH.

Abnormalities and management principles
- High lactate levels are more predictive of subsequent neurological disability than a low pH.
- Levels >4.2 mmol/L have been suggested as a trigger for delivery.

Management principles
- Early delivery of the fetus to avoid hypoxic injury when lactate levels exceed 4.2 mmol/L.

Limitations and complications
- Further work needed to ascertain validity of trigger values.
- May be nonhypoxic reasons for high lactate.

Test: Fetal electrocardiogram (ECG) analysis

Assessment of fetal well-being using electrodes attached to the fetal scalp once membranes ruptured. ECG analysis by computer specifically looking at ST changes, which may reflect hypoxia. The use of ST waveform analysis has been associated with neonates with severe metabolic acidosis at birth, fetal scalp blood sampling and operative deliveries.

Fetal well-being: Postnatal investigations

Test: Cord blood sampling

Indications
- Postpartum – assessment of hypoxia, acid-base balance or for research purposes.
- All caesarean sections, instrumental deliveries, meconium staining, deliveries where fetal scalp blood testing has been performed or if the neonatal condition is poor.
- Useful medicolegal tool.
- In pregnancy – investigation and diagnosis of fetal abnormality (as with fetal blood sampling and amniocentesis in utero).

How it is done
- A 10–20-cm segment of cord should be double clamped immediately after delivery to reduce erroneous alterations of pH and gas values resulting from continuing metabolism and gaseous diffusion.
- Postpartum samples must be taken from both umbilical artery and vein and promptly tested for pH, PO_2, PCO_2 and base excess.

Interpretation
Physiological principles
See arterial blood gas in Chapter 2, and Table 8.4.

Table 8.4 **Normal ranges in fetal cord sampling**

	Venous	Arterial
pH	7.20–7.41	7.15–7.38
PO_2 (kPa)	3.7–4.2	2.1–2.6
PCO_2 (kPa)	3.5–7.9	4.9–10.7
Base excess	0–5	0–10

Management principles
- Umbilical arterial (rather than venous) blood pH and gas values provide the best information on fetal acidosis.

- In association with APGAR scoring (see later) may be indicative of further hypoxia-related problems and may guide need for postnatal care.
- Can be used to distinguish hypoxia-induced low APGAR scores from non-hypoxia causes.
- Metabolic acidaemia is one of the essential criteria for establishing an intrapartum cause for cerebral palsy.
- Severe metabolic acidosis (pH <7.0–7.04) has been shown to correlate with neurological dysfunction and death. However the majority of neonates with pH <7.0 will be functionally normal.
- Cord PO_2 is not particularly useful as many newborns are initially hypoxaemic until normal extrauterine respiration is established.
- Respiratory acidosis alone is not predictive of long-term injury.
- Normal postpartum cord gases virtually exclude intrapartum cause for hypoxia-related problems.
- A difference of PCO_2 of >3.3 kPa indicates an acute rather than a chronic (prelabour) acidosis.
- Note that records need to be kept for 25 years for medicolegal purposes.

Limitations and complications
- An end-point that does not aid avoidance of hypoxia but only helps diagnosis.

Test: APGAR scoring

Indications
- All newborn babies.

How it is done
- Performed at 1 minute and 5 minutes after birth and assessing the newborn's status through muscle tone, heart rate, reflex response, colour and breathing. Scored 0–2 for each variable (Table 8.5).

Table 8.5 **APGAR data presented as**			
	0	1	2
Activity (muscle tone)	Limp; no movement	Some flexion of arms and legs	Active motion
Pulse (heart rate)	No heart rate	Fewer than 100 beats per minute	At least 100 beats per minute
Grimace (reflex response)	No response to airways being suctioned	Grimace during suctioning	Grimace and pull away, cough, or sneeze during suctioning
Appearance (colour)	The baby's whole body is completely bluish-grey or pale	Good colour in body with bluish hands or feet	Good colour all over
Respiration (breathing)	Not breathing	Weak cry; may sound like whimpering, slow or irregular breathing	Good, strong cry; normal rate and effort of breathing

Interpretation

Normal range

A score of 7 or above at 1 minute suggests good health.

Abnormalities and management principles

- Scores of 4–6 mean conservative measures such as suctioning or oxygen might be needed.
- 3 or below at 1 minute suggest problems. Call a paediatrician – interventions may be required such as tracheal intubation and/or resuscitation.
- Look for an improvement in scores to above 7 at 5 minutes.

Management principles

- Simple and repeatable bedside test.
- Nonspecific test for fetal depression (e.g. due to maternal drug effects, fetal anomalies, prematurity).
- Commonly low in premature infants, emergency caesarean sections.
- A low 1-minute score is not indicative of future problems.
- An APGAR of 0–3 at 5 minutes correlates with neonatal mortality but is not predictive of future neurological status.

Limitations and complications

- Poor predictive value for long-term outcome.
- Not useful in preterm infants.
- 75% of children with subsequent cerebral palsy had normal APGAR scores at 5 minutes.

Further investigations

- Cord blood sampling ascertains a hypoxic cause for low APGAR score.

Maternal well-being

Test: Electrocardiogram

Changes in the electrocardiogram (ECG) in pregnancy are due to alterations in ventricular mass and the position of the heart. The enlarging uterus causes upward movement of the diaphragm causing the heart to shift to the left and anteriorly. These changes result in left axis deviation and nonspecific ST segment changes. Flow murmurs are also common.

Test: Antenatal tests in the UK

- Blood group and antibody screen. It is recommended that routine antenatal anti-D prophylaxis be offered to all nonsensitized pregnant women who are RhD negative. Women should be screened for atypical red cell alloantibodies in early pregnancy and again at 28 weeks regardless of their RhD status. Haemoglobin levels outside the normal UK range for pregnancy (11 g/dL at first contact and 10.5 g/dL at 28 weeks) should be investigated and iron supplementation considered if indicated.
- Routine blood test include full blood count, urea and electrolytes, liver function tests and random glucose.
- Serological tests include rubella antibody status, syphilis, HIV and hepatitis B serology.
- Midstream urine.
- Screening for haemoglobinopathies.
- Obstetric ultrasound scan. Pregnant women should be offered an ultrasound scan to screen for structural anomalies and placental localization, ideally between 18 and 20 weeks' gestation.

Test: Blood tests during pregnancy

Renal function tests

Interpretation

- During pregnancy the serum sodium is about 3–5 mmol/L lower than normal because of an increase in intravascular volume.
- Cardiac output and renal blood flows are also increased.
- Glomerular filtration rate (GFR) is increased with resultant decrease in concentrations of serum urea, creatinine and uric acid.

Table 8.6 shows renal function values in pregnant and non-pregnant women.

Table 8.6 Renal function values in pregnant and nonpregnant women			
Electrolyte	Nonpregnant	Pregnant	Abnormalities
Sodium (mmol/L)	135–145	132–140	Depends on clinical state
Potassium (mmol/L)	3.5–5.5	3.2–4.6	Depends on clinical state
Creatinine (mmol/L)	0.06–0.1	0.04–0.08	Increased in: renal failure, pre-eclampsia
Urea (mmol/L)	2.5–6.8	1.0–3.8	Increased in: dehydration, pre-eclampsia (late stages), renal Impairment, hyperemesis gravidarum

Liver function tests

Interpretation

Physiological principles

- Serum albumin, transaminases (aspartate aminotransferase (AST) and alanine aminotransferase (ALT)) and total bilirubin are low compared with the non pregnant state due to the expansion of extracellular fluid (Table 8.7).
- Serum alkaline phosphatase (ALP) is elevated as it is secreted by the placenta.

Table 8.7 Comparison of liver enzymes between pregnant and nonpregnant			
Liver enzyme	Nonpregnant	Pregnant	Abnormalities
Albumin (g/L)	33–41	24–31	Increased in: Intrahepatic cholestasis of pregnancy HELLP Late stages of pre-eclampsia Acute fatty liver Viral hepatitides
AST (U/L)	1–30	1–21	As above
ALT (U/L)	1–40	1–30	As above
Bilirubin (mol/L)	3–22	3–14	As above
Alkaline phosphatase (U/L)	25–100	125–250	Increased in metabolic bone disorders (when placental serum ALP excluded)

The use of electronic fetal monitoring: the use and interpretation of cardiotocography in intrapartum fetal surveillance. Published May 2001 by the Royal College of Obstetricians and Gynaecologists. http://www.rcog.org.uk

Platelet count

Platelet count may be reduced by:

- Pregnancy-induced causes (e.g. pre-eclampsia, gestational thrombocytopaenia, **h**aemolysis **e**levated **l**iver enzymes **l**ow **p**latelet (HELLP) syndrome)
- Non-pregnancy-related causes (e.g. infection, immune thrombocytopaenic purpura, leukaemia, etc.).

In a normal pregnancy platelet count may be reduced, whilst in pre-eclampsia there may be a reduction in platelet function as well as number. There is limited data to suggest a safe lower limit for regional blockade. In our institution, an isolated platelet count of $>80 \times 10^9$/L is acceptable for siting a regional block. An isolated platelet count between 50 and 80×10^9/L should be discussed with a haematologist and an obstetric anaesthetist. Consider the use of the TEG (thromboelastography) or PFA-100 (platelet function analyzer). A platelet count of $<50 \times 10^9$/L is an absolute contraindication to a regional block.

TOPIC ❾

Intensive care

Topic Contents

Cardiac output monitoring 165
Test: Pulmonary artery catheter **165**
Test: Oesophageal Doppler monitor (ODM) **167**
Test: Lithium dilution cardiac output (LiDCO plus) **168**
Test: Pulse-induced contour cardiac output (PiCCO) **170**
Test: Noninvasive cardiac output (NICO) monitor **170**
Test: Impedance cardiography **171**
Test: Echocardiography **171**
Perioperative optimization 171
Test: Central venous pressure (CVP) **172**

Test: Invasive arterial pressure monitoring **173**
Monitors of organ perfusion 174
Indication **174**
Test: Serum lactate **174**
Test: Base deficit **175**
Test: Anion gap **175**
Test: Mixed venous oxygen saturation (SvO$_2$) **176**
Test: Gastric tonometry and the CO$_2$ gap **177**
Other investigations performed in intensive care 177
Test: Intra-abdominal pressure (IAP) **177**
Test: Ultrasound in intensive care **178**

Cardiac output monitoring

Indications

1. To aid management of patients with haemodynamic instability. This may be in the setting of isolated cardiac dysfunction, e.g. myocardial infarction or acute left ventricular failure; more often in critically ill patients there is combined pathology – hypovolaemia and distributive shock as well as associated cardiac dysfunction. Rationalizing appropriate vasoconstrictor, inodilator and fluid therapy is enhanced with knowledge of cardiovascular parameters.
2. To aid management of surgical patients at high risk due to intrinsic cardiac disease or other comorbidities. Cardiac output (CO) monitoring instituted in the perioperative period with goal-directed therapy has a growing body of clinical evidence of outcome benefit.

Method

New technology has resulted in a number of techniques, which range vary in invasiveness (Table 9.1).

Test: Pulmonary artery catheter

- Considered by many to be the gold standard of cardiac output monitoring.
- Position less assured with advent of newer techniques and uncertainty of outcome benefit in addition to suggestion of possible harm.

Table 9.1 **Invasiveness of monitoring methods**		
Invasive	**Moderately invasive**	**Noninvasive**
Pulmonary artery catheter	ODM LIDCO PICCO NICO TOE	Impedance cardiography (ICG) Transthoracic echocardiography

- Balloon-tipped catheter is floated through right heart and 'wedged' in medium-sized pulmonary artery.
- Thermodilution principle is used to measure CO using preterminal thermistor.
- Two methods:
  - Cold injectate – 10 mL normal saline or 5% dextrose solution (cold or room temperature) injected quickly through proximal port produces a temperature change in blood detected by thermistor. Area under curve of resultant temperature/time curve (Fig. 9.1) is inversely proportional to CO. Usually averaged over three measurements at end-expiration.
  - Continuous cardiac output – uses same principle, but uses pulses of heat from a filament to produce the temperature/time curve.

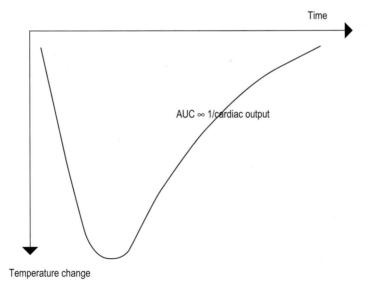

Fig. 9.1 Cold injectate temperature change. Area under curve inversely proportional to Cardiac Output.

Provides information regarding pulmonary as well as systemic vasculature.

- Measured variables (normal values in brackets):
  - Right atrial pressure (5–8 mmHg)
  - Pulmonary artery pressure (systolic 15–25 mmHg, diastolic 8–15 mmHg)
  - Pulmonary artery occlusion pressure (PAOP) (6–15 mmHg)
  - Cardiac output – derived via Stewart Hamilton method (4–7 L/minute)
  - Mixed venous oxygen saturation (SvO_2) drawn from distal port (70–75%) – see below.
- Calculated variables:
  - Stroke volume (60–100 mL/beat, varies with age)
  - Systemic vascular resistance (SVR) (1000–1500 dyne s/cm^5)
  - Pulmonary vascular resistance (PVR) (<250 dyne s/cm^5).

Interpretation

- PAOP low in hypovolaemia, raised due to left ventricular failure or mitral valve disease.
- Low SVR represents vasodilated state, high suggests vasoconstriction.
- CO low may reflect hypovolaemia or impaired cardiac function, CO is raised in hyperdynamic states (e.g. sepsis, thyrotoxicosis, inotrope therapy).

Limitations

- Invasive
- Requires technical skills
- Arrhythmias result in unreliable data
- Risk of:
  - catheter-related infection (limit placement to maximum 72 hours)
  - Pulmonary infarction if continuously wedged
  - Potential damage to cardiac and pulmonary structures (NB always deflate balloon prior to withdrawing catheter).

Test: Oesophageal Doppler monitor (ODM)

- Flexible ultrasound probe placed in distal oesophagus under anaesthesia/sedation via mouth or nose and focused to produce a Doppler waveform trace corresponding to flow of blood in descending aorta (Fig. 9.2).

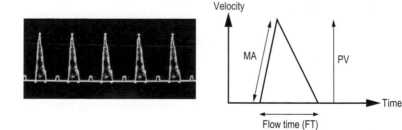

Fig. 9.2 OCM waveform.

- Softer flexible nasal probes available for awake patients.
- Doppler ultrasound is used to quantify velocity of blood in descending aorta during systole.
- Combining this with estimated aortic cross-sectional area gives the stroke volume.
- Stroke volume × heart rate = cardiac output.

- Flow time (FT) represents systolic time and is corrected (FT_c) to a heart rate of 60 bpm with a further correction factor for the unmeasured upper extremity blood flow (i.e. carotid/subclavian flow).
- Measured variables: Mean acceleration.
- Calculated variables: Stroke volume, peak velocity (PV), cardiac output, flow time, systemic vascular resistance.

Interpretation

Based on pattern recognition using all the indices. Using one single parameter should not be relied upon for decision making (normal values in brackets):

- FT_c (330–360 ms) – reduced in hypovolaemia and vasoconstriction. High values may represent cardiac failure or vasodilatation in a volume replete patient.
- PV (varies with age, lower limit of normal approximately 120 − age) – marker of contractility.
- MA ($10–12 \text{ m/s}^2$) – affected primarily by contractility.
- SV – low values occur in hypovolaemia, cardiac failure, increased afterload.

Contraindications and limitations

- Pharyngo-oesophageal pathology.
- Presence of intra-aortic balloon pump (IABP) makes data unreliable.
- No pulmonary data obtained.
- Difficult to interpret with arrhythmias.
- User variability in focusing probe.

Suprasternal Doppler

- Similar principle to ODM, however ultrasound signal probe placed in suprasternal notch to measure flow in aortic arch.
- Direction of probe manipulated to achieve best audible signal and trace.
- Not widely used partly due to concerns of reproducibility of measured results.

Test: Lithium dilution cardiac output (LiDCO plus)

- Lithium chloride injected as a bolus via central (ideally) or peripheral line.
- Blood is drawn from an arterial line, past a lithium sensor producing a lithium concentration/time curve.
- Mathematical application to the area under this curve provides an estimate of cardiac output.
- Pulse power cardiac output software (Pulse CO) uses this information to calibrate the arterial waveform such that each pulse is a quantified estimate of the patient's stroke volume (Fig. 9.3).
- Hence provides 'beat to beat' (time averaged) cardiac output monitoring.
- Also has the facility to quantify the pulse pressure variation (PPV), systolic pressure variation (SPV) and stroke volume variation (SVV) – each providing preload status information.
- Calculates oxygen delivery (DO_2).

Limitations

- Contraindicated in lithium therapy.
- Stroke volume variation interpretation difficult with arrhythmias.
- Pregnancy (first trimester).
- Regular recalibration recommended.
- Muscle paralysis affects calibration.

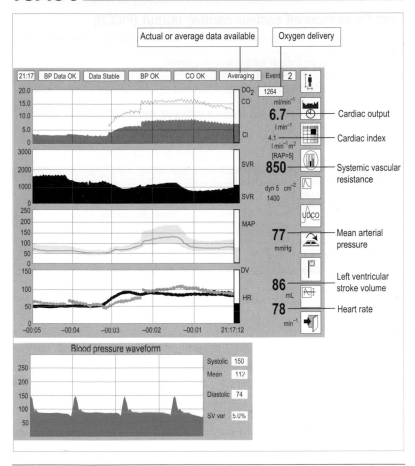

Fig. 9.3 Pulse power cardiac output software (Pulse CO) display.

- Requires arterial +/− central access.
- Aortic valve regurgitation will cause inaccuracies.
- Excessive positive end-expiratory pressure (PEEP) will overestimate SVV.
- Intra-aortic balloon pump affects data.

Interpretation

- CO/SV/SVR as above.
- SVV, PPV, SPV values above 10% suggest hypovolaemia, predicting fluid responsiveness in the *fully mechanically* ventilated patient.
- DO_2 (850–1200 mL/minute): low values suggest hypovolaemia, low cardiac output, hypoxaemia or anaemia. Raised with hyperdynamic state.

Test: Pulse-induced contour cardiac output (PiCCO)

- Some similarities to cold injectate thermodilution pulmonary artery catheter (PAC) and LIDCO method.
- Bolus injectate given through *central venous catheter*.
- Thermistor at tip of centrally placed arterial catheter – femoral (usual), brachial or axillary.
- *Transpulmonary* thermodilution curve produced and modified Stewart-Hamilton method applied to calculate cardiac output.
- Pulse contour analysis (Table 9.2) applies a calibrated algorithm to calculate the stroke volume from each pulse wave.
- Further mathematical algorithms are applied to obtain other volumetric parameters (listed).

Table 9.2 **Variables in monitoring contour cardiac output**	
Thermodilution variables	**Pulse contour variables**
Cardiac output	Continuous cardiac output
Global end-diastolic volume index (GEDI)	Sytemic vascular resistance
Extravascular lung water index (ELWI)	Stroke volume
Intrathoracic blood volume index (ITBI)	dP/dtmax
Global ejection fraction (GEF)	Stroke volume/pulse pressure variation
Cardiac function index (CFI)	
Pulmonary vascular permeabilty index (PVPI)	

Interpretation (normal values in brackets)

- CO/SV/SVR/SVV/PVV as above.
- Global end-diastolic volume index (GEDI) (680–800 mL/m^2). Represents volume of blood in the heart.
- Extravascular lung water. (ELWI (3–7 mL/kg). Water content of lungs, i.e. degree of pulmonary oedema (cardio- or noncardiogenic). If raised then further volume loading may lead to deterioration in oxygenation.
- Pulmonary vascular permeability index (PVPI) (1–3.0). May suggest aetiology of pulmonary oedema. High values consistent with increased capillary permeability, i.e. noncardiogenic, normal values suggest cardiogenic origin.
- GEF/CFI/dP$_{max}$ – markers of contractility.

Contraindications/limitations:

- Requires regular recalibration (8-hourly)
- Central access and large arterial access required
- Some parameters difficult to interpret with arrhythmias
- IABP makes data interpretation difficult
- Erroneous results with aortic aneurysms when using femoral thermistor.

Test: Noninvasive cardiac output (NICO) monitor

- Requires tracheal intubation
- Consists of a microprocessor system (connected to patient via ET tube) measuring end-tidal CO_2 partial pressure, ($P_{ET}CO_2$) and calculating the total CO_2 elimination over a respiratory cycle (VCO_2).

- System set up to allow intermittent partial rebreathing of CO_2 for periods of 35 seconds by increasing dead space every 3 minutes.
- Rebreathing results in higher alveolar CO_2 ($P_{ET}CO_2$) and overall decreased CO_2 elimination (VCO_2).
- Extrapolation of Fick principle suggests ratio of ΔVCO_2 and $\Delta P_{ET}CO_2$ is proportional to cardiac output.
- Data provided: Cardiac output, SpO_2, tidal volume, $ETCO_2$, VCO_2, dead space volume, respiratory rate, pulse rate, airway pressure.

Limitations

- Only applicable to ventilated patients.
- Blood flow through shunt area (Q_s) is not incorporated into calculation. Instead Q_s is estimated from SpO_2 and subsequently added.
- May overestimate CO in spontaneously breathing patients.

Test: Impedance cardiography

- Small current applied across thorax via four dual sensor electrodes on neck and chest.
- Impedance (resistance) to current measured.
- Impedance changes proportional to volume/flow of blood in thorax.
- Thoracic blood volume changes with each cardiac contraction.
- Mathematical modelling allows estimation of cardiac output from subsequent impedance change curves.
- Not widely used partly due to concerns regarding assumptions made in mathematical derivation affecting accuracy.
- There is increasing clinical evidence supporting its use with promising applications in critically ill patients.

Test: Echocardiography

- Transthoracic or transoesophageal.
- Two-dimensional ultrasound visualization of ventricular chamber estimates volume at end diastole and systole.
- Difference between systolic and diastolic volume equates to stroke volume (see Chapter 3 for more information).
- Also able to assess ventricular function and reveal related pathology, e.g. pericardial effusion, regional wall motion abnormality, valvular lesions and estimate pulmonary artery pressure.

Limitations

- Specialist skills required.
- Noncontinuous data.
- Potential for oesophageal injury with TOE.

Perioperative optimization

- Goal-directed therapy as distinct from *resuscitation* of ill patients prior to surgery.
- Patients able to mount a cardiovascular response to major surgery and achieve particular goals, i.e. cardiac index >4.5 L/minute/m^2 and tissue oxygen delivery >600 mL/minute/m^2 have a better outcome in the perioperative period.

- Manipulation of a patient's physiology to match these parameters is the cornerstone of optimization.
- Mounting clinical evidence that this confers a positive outcome in the perioperative period.
- Ideally goals targeted preoperatively, but can be done with benefit intra- or postoperatively.
- Advent of noninvasive cardiac output monitors described above has made assessing the goals much easier.
- Well known physiological equations applied:
  - $CI = CO/BSA$
  - $DO_2I = CI \times$ oxygen content of arterial blood (CaO_2)
  - $CaO_2 = 1.34 \times Hb \times$ arterial saturation/100.
- Therefore parameters that can be manipulated are:
  - SaO_2 – supplemental oxygen/ventilation (aim >95%)
  - Cardiac output – fluid therapy/cardiac inotropes (aim >4.5 L/minute/m^2)
  - Haemoglobin – blood transfusion (aim 8–10 g/dL).
- Evidence suggests that if goal-directed therapy is to be initiated postoperatively, targets should be met within the first hour and continued for 8 hours post op.

Test: Central venous pressure (CVP)

Indications
1. To guide fluid resuscitation.
2. Management of heart failure.
3. Drug administration (e.g. inotropes, parenteral nutrition).

Method
- Catheter can be placed via internal jugular (commonest), subclavian, femoral or antecubital vein approach.
- Multi lumen lines are inserted using Seldinger technique. Single lumen lines may be sited using Seldinger or catheter over needle method.
- NICE guidelines (2002) recommend use of 2D ultrasound to guide catheter placement particularly via internal jugular route (see Chapter 3 for more information on this technique). Otherwise landmark method used.
- Correct *thoracic* placement should be confirmed with a chest x-ray, showing the catheter within the SVC and the tip at the level of the tracheal carina. Waveform and blood gas analysis (although acceptable for femoral cannulation) will only confirm venous intrathoracic placement and not position.
- Measurements represent right atrial pressure and hence right ventricular end diastolic pressure (RVEDP).
- Commonly (and mistakenly) taken to represent preload, however preload is a function of right ventricular end diastolic volume (RVEDV) not RVEDP, which will be dependent on compliance of ventricle.
- Preload assessed by dynamic changes in response to a fluid challenge (see below).
- Assuming normal anatomy and structure of heart and lungs this will also represent left heart pressure.

Interpretation
- CVP: (normal range 6–12 mmHg). Static measurement less helpful in guiding fluid resuscitation since compliance of right heart will affect reading for any given RVEDV. Dynamic measurements with response to fluid challenges are more informative – see below. In the context of left ventricular failure higher values are more reliable since they reflect poorly compliant ventricle and 'off loading' (diuresis/venodilatation) may be appropriate.

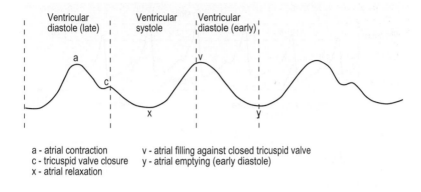

a - atrial contraction
c - tricuspid valve closure
x - atrial relaxation

v - atrial filling against closed tricuspid valve
y - atrial emptying (early diastole)

Fig. 9.4 CVP trace: right atrial pressure.

- Waveform interpretation (see Fig. 9.4)
  - Tricuspid regurgitation: CV waves.
  - Tricuspid or pulmonary stenosis: giant a waves
  - Complete heart block, junctional rhythm, VT: cannon a waves
  - Atrial fibrillation: absent a waves

Fluid challenge
Assess response to fast 250 mL fluid bolus:
- CVP rises then falls over 10 minutes with overall increase <3 mmHg – underfilled
- CVP rises then equilibrates at a value between 3 and 5 mmHg above baseline – optimal
- CVP rises and equilibrates 5 mmHg above baseline – fluid overload, further fluid may result in pulmonary oedema.

Test: Invasive arterial pressure monitoring

Indications
1. Monitoring patients with actual or potential cardiovascular instability.
2. Monitoring patients receiving inotropic/vasoconstrictor support.
3. Situations necessitating strict arterial pressure goals, e.g. head injury/cerebral oedema.
4. Patients receiving ventilatory support or requiring frequent arterial blood gas analysis.
5. To allow repeated assessment of metabolic abnormalities, e.g. acidaemia, lactataemia.

Method
- 20 G or 22 G catheter sited in artery.
- Most commonly sited in radial artery due to lower complication rates – brachial and femoral arteries are other common sites.
- 'Allen test' should ideally be performed prior to insertion to identify competent ulnar artery blood flow.
- Each pulse is transmitted through a column of fluid (usually heparinized saline) under pressure, within optimally compliant tubing, to a transducer which converts this to give a waveform and numerical data.
- The transducer should be placed at the level of the heart, unless managing head injured patients, when it may be 'zeroed' at level of mastoid.
- Transducer system pressurized to stop blood passing beyond catheter into tubing and flushed ~4 mL/hour to ensure patency.

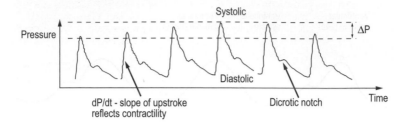

Fig. 9.5 Arterial trace.

Interpretation
See Fig. 9.5.
- Systolic/diastolic/mean arterial pressure.
- dp/dt – steep upstroke represents increased cardiac contractility against low systemic vascular resistance.
- Dicrotic notch – occurs low in vasodilatation and high in vasoconstriction (NB position also shifts higher the more central the artery is catheterized).
- ΔP –systolic pressure variation. Values greater than 10 mmHg may suggest hypovolaemia.
- Pulse pressure is the systolic minus the diastolic pressure. Low in aortic stenosis. High in aortic regurgitation and sepsis.
- Area within pulse wave proportional to stroke volume.

Contraindications/limitations
- Limb ischaemia.
- Care with anticoagulated patients.
- Avoid ulnar artery.
- Measurements may be unreliable if trace not optimally 'damped' to ensure no over or under reading.

Monitors of organ perfusion

Indication
- Although monitors of cardiac output can tell us whether oxygen is being delivered to the tissues, they cannot tell us whether that oxygen is being utilized. Failure to utilize oxygen may be due to inadequate delivery at a global or microcirculatory level, or may be due to mitochondrial failure at a cellular level, such as that seen with severe sepsis.
- Monitors of perfusion can help indicate whether a problem of oxygen delivery or utilization exists, and help monitor it.
- Clinical monitors of perfusion adequacy include conscious level and urine output. In addition, capillary refill time and core–peripheral temperature difference may be used. However, all these clinical signs are susceptible to changes independent of perfusion, and hence lack specificity.
- Biochemical markers of global perfusion adequacy may be more sensitive and specific.

Test: Serum lactate
- Under normal conditions, glucose is broken down to pyruvate, yielding two molecules of ATP via anaerobic glycolysis. Pyruvate then enters the Krebs cycle within the mitochondrion, undergoing aerobic glycolysis to yield a further 32 molecules of ATP. This process requires oxygen.

- Lactate is formed from pyruvate under conditions where there is insufficient oxygen for pyruvate to enter the Krebs cycle, and thus may act as a monitor of oxygenation at a cellular level.
- Normal serum level is <2 mmol/L, being produced at a rate of approximately 0.8 mmol/kg/hour, a testament to the enormous capacity to metabolize lactate by the liver, skeletal muscle, kidneys and brain.
- A serum level >4 mmol/L is associated with a poor outcome in severe sepsis. However, there are many other causes of an increased lactate, and thus careful interpretation of an elevated lactate is necessary to rule these out (see Table 9.3).

Test: Base deficit

- If the serum lactate cannot be measured, an assessment of the metabolic component of any acidosis seen on arterial blood gas analysis can give an important estimate of the degree of perfusion inadequacy. The base excess provides such an assessment.
- It is equivalent to the amount of base required to normalize the pH of a sample of patient's blood, under standard conditions (a temperature of $37°C$ and, most importantly, a normal pCO_2 of 5.3 kPa (40 mmHg), to exclude any respiratory component of the acidosis).
- A high base deficit implies that the main physiological buffer, HCO_3^-, has been lost, either to neutralize excess acid production (e.g. lactate, ketones, or sulphate in renal failure), or it has been lost directly via the kidneys (renal tubular acidosis) or GI tract (diarrhoea, ureteric diversion).
- To differentiate between these two classes of metabolic acidosis, calculation of the anion gap is required.
- Base deficit can be classified according to severity:
  - Mild 2–5 mmol/L
  - Moderate 6–14 mmol/L
  - Severe >15 mmol/L.
- A base deficit of 6 mmol/L or more has been shown to be a marker of injury severity and a poor prognostic indicator.

Test: Anion gap

- As well as lactate, a number of other metabolic acids are produced during ischaemic states.
- Their presence in increased amounts can be deduced via calculation of the anion gap, which represents the difference between measured strong cations (Na^+, K^+) and strong anions (Cl^-, HCO_3^-).
- Because electroneutrality must be maintained, this difference is made up of unmeasured weak anions such as albumin, phosphate and metabolic acids, and is usually in the range of 8–16 mmol/L, depending on the albumin concentration.

Table 9.3 Causes of a raised lactate

Global tissue ischaemia –	Shock, sepsis
Regional tissue ischaemia –	Gut ischaemia, compartment syndrome
Mitochondrial inability to utilize oxygen –	Severe sepsis, CO/CN poisoning
Reduced elimination –	Primary liver disease/reduced hepatic blood flow
Compounds that affect lactate metabolism –	Ketones, Metformin
Increased metabolic rate –	Adrenaline, Salbutamol
Other compounds metabolized to lactate –	Ethanol, methanol
Increased production by skeletal muscles –	Exercise, fitting

Table 9.4 **Common causes of a raised anion gap**
Lactate acidosis
Ketoacidosis
Renal failure
Drug overdose – particularly salicylates
Toxins – methanol, ethylene glycol

- If the concentration of metabolic acid increases due to inadequate perfusion, the anion gap will also increase (see Table 9.4).

Test: Mixed venous oxygen saturation (SvO_2)

Indications
- As a surrogate marker of cardiac output and tissue oxygenation.
- As an endpoint in resuscitation.

How it is done
- The mixed venous oxygen saturation (SvO_2) represents the saturation of blood in the pulmonary artery, sampled from the distal tip of a pulmonary artery catheter.
- In practice, a blood sample from the distal lumen of a central line may be taken. This does not require the insertion of a pulmonary artery catheter and represents the central venous oxygen saturation – $ScvO_2$ (see below).
- Alternatively a central venous catheter that continuously monitors central venous oxygen saturation ($ScvO_2$) may be used.

Interpretation
- Values represent the balance between oxygen content and cardiac output (supply/delivery) and extraction (demand/consumption).
- Under constant oxygen content, changes in SvO_2 reflect the relation between whole body oxygen consumption and cardiac output.
- The saturation is normally between 70% and 75%. A normal SvO_2 can help to confirm that oxygen delivery (and its primary determinant, cardiac output) is adequate for the body's total oxygen requirements and hence that perfusion is adequate. A reduced SvO_2 represents:
  - Reduction in oxygen delivery, due to either a fall in cardiac output or a drop in haemoglobin concentration
  - An increased oxygen consumption due to an increase in metabolic rate (e.g. caused by sepsis, thyrotoxicosis).
- An increased SvO_2 represents tissue shunting or inadequate oxygen utilization, for example in some forms of sepsis, cirrhosis or arteriovenous shunting. It can also point to overdose of inotropic support.

Physiological principles
- SvO_2 is a far more sensitive indicator of likely perfusion inadequacy than routine haemodynamic measurements such as heart rate and blood pressure. However, it requires accurate placement of a PA catheter, which may be quite difficult.
- A surrogate measure that is frequently used instead is the mixed central venous oxygen saturation ($ScvO_2$), which represents the saturation of venous blood sampled from the superior vena cava (SVC), via the distal lumen of a central venous catheter.
- Although changes in $ScvO_2$ broadly track changes in SvO_2 in both health and illness, the exact relationship between the two values is complex. In health, the SvO_2 is slightly higher

than the ScvO$_2$ because of the high oxygen consumption of the brain, compared to the rest of the body (ScvO$_2$ represents venous drainage from the head and upper body). During shock states, however, there is physiological diversion of blood from the gut in an attempt to optimize oxygen delivery to more vital organs, making venous blood from the GI tract more desaturated.

- Thus, the ScvO$_2$, which does not incorporate this desaturated venous blood, will have a higher value than the SvO$_2$, which does.

Management principles

- There is evidence that increasing ScvO$_2$ to more than 70% (in addition to other measures) with fluids, blood and inotropes/vasoactive drugs lowers mortality in an early sepsis.

Limitations

- For correct interpretation of SvO$_2$, it is preferable that arterial oxygen saturation is >97%.
- Being a global measure, however, a normal value cannot exclude the presence of regional hypoperfusion, e.g. gut ischaemia.
- A normal or high SvO$_2$ does not rule out pathological oxygen delivery, for example in peripheral shunting in sepsis due to inadequate oxygen utilization in the tissues.
- Requires insertion of a PA catheter (ScvO$_2$) or central venous line (SvO$_2$).

Test: Gastric tonometry and the CO$_2$ gap

- In the early stages of shock, one of the compensatory mechanisms to maintain oxygen delivery to vital organs is the diversion of blood away from less essential organs such as the gut.
- This may cause anaerobic respiration in the gastrointestinal (GI) tract wall, and a commensurate acidosis. The additional H$^+$ ions are buffered by HCO$_3$ to form CO$_2$.
- This increase in CO$_2$ within the GI tract wall equilibrates with the GI tract lumen, and can be detected using a gastric tonometer. This is essentially a saline-filled balloon, which sits within the stomach.
- The CO$_2$ tension within the stomach lumen equilibrates with the saline, which is then repeatedly aspirated and analyzed using a CO$_2$ sensor connected to the tonometry tube. The difference between the gastric CO$_2$ tension and arterial CO$_2$ tension (termed 'the CO$_2$ gap') will be proportional to the degree of gut ischaemia present.
- Normal values are 15–20 kPa.
- Although this technique has shown efficacy in many small trials, it has yet to be demonstrated in a large, randomized controlled trial that measurement and correction of the CO$_2$ gap improves mortality. However, prevention of the development of a large CO$_2$ gap intraoperatively, by optimizing haemodynamics in an attempt to maintain GI tract perfusion, has been shown to improve perioperative morbidity in certain surgical subgroups.

Other investigations performed in intensive care

Test: Intra-abdominal pressure (IAP)

- The pressure within the abdominal cavity is normally 5–7 mmHg.
- In critically ill patients IAP may exceed this.
- Intra-abdominal hypertension (IAH) is defined as IAP $\geq$12 mmHg and graded as shown in Table 9.5.
- Abdominal compartment syndrome is defined as sustained IAP >20 mmHg associated with new organ dysfunction.
- May be primary (pathology within the abdomen and/or pelvis) or secondary (extra-abdominal pathology).

Table 9.5 **Grades of intra-abdominal hypertension**

Grade	Intra-abdominal pressure (mmHg)
I	12–15
II	16–20
III	21–25
IV	>25

Method

- Most common technique involves measuring bladder pressure.
- Urinary catheter placed within bladder of supine patient *lying flat*.
- 25 mL of sterile saline instilled into bladder with catheter tubing clamped at distal end.
- A pressure transducer is inserted via the sampling port of the catheter and zeroed level with the symphysis pubis.
- Numerous commercial kits available. Alternatively after clamping, the catheter tubing can be held vertically at right angles to the patient and used as a manometer. The height of the meniscus gives IAP in cmH_2O (1 mmHg $=$ 1.36 cmH_2O).
- End expiratory value taken.

Test: Ultrasound in intensive care

Indications

- Improving line placement safety.
- Aiding insertion of tracheostomy.
- Evaluating haemodynamics using echocardiography (see Chapter 3).
- Diagnosis and drainage of intrathoracic and intra-abdominal fluid collections.
- Trauma: the FAST examination (see Chapter 2).

Diagnosis of deep vein thrombosis. For a more detailed description of the mechanism of ultrasound, refer to Chapter 3.

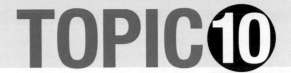

TOPIC ⑩
Therapeutic drug monitoring

Topic Contents

Introduction 179
Gentamicin 180
Digoxin 180
Phenytoin 180

Theophylline/aminophylline 184
Vancomycin 184
Commonly prescribed drugs needing TDM 184

Introduction

Drugs that are suitable for therapeutic drug monitoring (TDM) have a recognized desired serum concentration range. Within this range the drug will produce its optimal effect with minimal toxicity. TDM is thus necessary for two reasons:

1. To determine the drug is at therapeutic plasma concentrations: for most drugs, the easiest way to determine efficacy is by achieving a clinical endpoint. However for certain drugs, TDM is the only way to ensure the drug is working.
2. To determine if the drug is at toxic levels: some drugs have a 'narrow therapeutic range', where the difference between efficacious and toxic concentrations is small. TDM aids drug dosing, keeping plasma levels within the desired efficacious range and out of the toxic range.

The drugs most likely to require TDM are gentamicin, vancomycin, phenytoin, digoxin and theophylline/aminophylline. When considering measuring a drug level, the following needs to be known.

Indication for TDM

- This may include achieving a therapeutic target, trying to avoid the toxic range, or both.
- Possible drug interaction. The drugs mentioned are prone to multiple drug interactions in relation to enzyme induction and inhibition.
- Change in renal or hepatic function. The drugs mentioned above are either renally excreted (gentamicin) or hepatically metabolized (phenytoin, digoxin, theophylline).

When to measure the drug level

Drug levels need to be taken at specific times to make sense of the results. It takes about 4–5 half-lives for a regularly administered drug to accumulate in the blood, at which point the drug is said to be in steady state. Ideally, one would wait for the drug to reach steady state before taking a level, but in the acute situation this luxury is not possible. Ideally before the drug has reached steady state, one should take one of the following:

- Trough level, i.e. sample immediately before the dose is due, when the drug concentration is at its lowest; or

- Peak level: timing depends on the half-life of a drug – the longer the distribution half-life, the longer the time before the drug concentration is at its highest.

Interpretation

The sample needs to be labelled with the time of sampling and the time of dosing. Without it, the result will be uninterpretable.

How to act on what you find

This is not always simple. When in doubt, get help! But before considering anything complex, ask yourself some simple questions:

- Was the patient compliant in the community?
- Is there a possible drug interaction?

If possible, find an alternative to the offending drug. If there is no alternative, but the offending drug is for a short course (e.g. an antibiotic), continue both drugs, monitor for signs of drug failure or toxicity and recheck levels when the offending drug is stopped. If there is no alternative, but the offending drug is needed for a more chronic duration, seek advice.

Gentamicin

There are two methods of gentamicin dosing, the 'conventional' method and the 'once-daily' method (Table 10.1). 'Once-daily' is extremely dangerous if used in patients with renal dysfunction, for this reason, some units only use 'conventional' dosing.

For obese patients, use corrected body weight:
- Ideal body weight (IBW) in kilograms:
  - –IBW (male) = 50 kg in weight + (2.3 × every inch over 5 ft in height)
  - –IBW (female) = 45 kg in weight + (2.3 × every inch over 5 ft in height)
- Excess body weight (EBW):

$$EBW \ (kg) = actual \ body \ weight - IBW$$

$$\% \ Obesity = \frac{actual \ body \ weight - IBW \times 100}{IBW}$$

- Corrected body weight (CBW):

$$CBW \ (kg) = IBW + (0.4 \times EBW)$$

Use if patient is >15% obese.

Digoxin

See Table 10.2 for the dosing regimen, and Box 10.1 for drugs that can increase or reduce levels of the drug.

Phenytoin

See Table 10.3 for the dosing regimen, and Box 10.2 for drugs that can increase or reduce levels of the drug.

Table 10.1 Gentamicin dosing regimens

Conventional dosing	1–1.5 mg/kg IV with frequency depending on estimated creatinine clearance (CrCl). If CrCl: • >70 mL/minute, 8-hourly • 30–70 mL/minute, 12-hourly • 10–30 mL/minute, 24-hourly • 5–10 mL/minute, 48-hourly
Indication	Avoid toxicity (trough) and efficacy (peak)
How it is done	Take a peak and trough level before the third dose or on day 2
Target	The trough level should be <2 mg/mL. The peak should be 4–8 mg/mL
Interpretation	If the trough level is >2 mg/mL, withhold the next doses until the level falls to <2 mg/mL Adjust the dosage interval rather than the actual dose If the peak is too low consult a pharmacist or microbiologist for advice
Once-daily dosing	7 mg/kg IV If obese, do not use their actual weight, but calculate their corrected body weight
Contraindication	Once-daily dosing is not appropriate for a CrCl <20 mL/minute, oliguria, haemofiltration, endocarditis, severe liver disease, cystic fibrosis, major burns, prophylaxis or infants <6 months
Indication	For safe and effective therapy
How it is done	Levels any time between 6 and 14 hours postdose
Interpretation	Refer to the Hartford nomogram (Fig. 10.1) If the levels are high, increase the interval between doses as per the Hartford nomogram

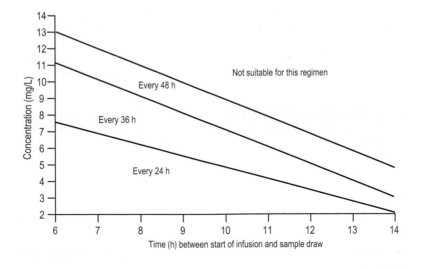

Fig. 10.1 Hartford nomogram for gentamicin once-daily dosing regimen.

Table 10.2 **Digoxin dosing regimen**

Loading dose	*Urgent:* 750 µg to 1 mg IV over 2 hours or 1–1.5 mg PO over 24 hours in divided doses (6-hourly loading allows for distribution and less nausea) *Less urgent:* 250–500 µg PO daily for 3 days
Maintenance dose	125–250 µg PO OD Less in the elderly or the renally impaired
Indication	Avoid toxicity Investigate treatment failure
How it is done	Take levels 1 week after starting treatment Sample 6–9 hours postdose, or immediately predose Not necessary in all patients starting therapy. Advisable in the elderly and the renally impaired
Interpretation	Recommended therapeutic range: • 0.5–0.8 µg/L (0.6–1 nanomol/L) target in heart failure • 1.5–2 µg/L (1.9–2.6 nanomol/L) target in arrhythmias >3 µg/L (3.8 nanomol/L) is usually associated with signs of toxicity Toxicity possible at levels as low as 1.5 µg/L (1.9 nanomol/L)
Action	**Patient toxic and levels raised:** • If life-threatening, i.e. level >4 µg/L (5.1 mol/L), omit drug, treat with Digibind (expensive) • Determine cause before restarting • If restarting, consider a lower dose. In general, to achieve a serum concentration of half the value, reduce the maintenance dose by half **Patient toxic but levels within therapeutic range:** • Exclude other causes of toxic symptoms • Check K$^+$ • Reduce dose, consider additional therapy for cardiac failure of arrhythmia **Patient clinically undertreated, and levels low:** • Increase dose, usually by 50–75 µg daily, and recheck levels **Patient clinically undertreated, but levels within therapeutic range:** • Consider additional therapy
Important	Hypokalaemia and hypothyroidism are commonly associated with digoxin toxicity, so in suspected toxicity check K$^+$ and thyroid function!

Box 10.1 **Drugs that affect digoxin levels in the body**

Can *increase* levels	Can *reduce* levels
Amiodarone	Antacids
Bendroflumethiazide	Cholestyramine
Ciclosporin	St John's Wort
Diltiazem	
Furosemide	
Itraconazole	
Macrolides	
Propafenone	

Box 10.1 **Continued**
Quinidine
Spironolactone
Telmisartan
Verapamil

Table 10.3 **Phenytoin dosing regimen**	
Loading dose	**15 mg/kg IV: maximum rate of 50 mg/minute**
Maintenance dose	100 mg IV 6- to 8-hourly 150–300 mg PO OD. Gradually increasing to 200–500 mg PO OD Doses can be split if not tolerated
Indication	Ensure achieving therapeutic target Avoid toxicity Narrow therapeutic index A fit free patient, with no signs of toxicity, requires no levels
How it is done	Steady state takes 2–4 weeks after starting the drug or changing the dose. In the acute ICU setting take daily levels *For IV regimen:* loading dose 2–4 hours to assess peak, otherwise predose sampling *For PO regimen:* trough level predose In an emergency, take levels at any time
Interpretation	Recommended therapeutic range 40–80 μmol/L or 10–20 mg/L Phenytoin is largely albumin bound, so in apparent hypoalbuminaemia, an apparently therapeutic level may actually be toxic. Hypoalbuminaemia will lead to an increased fraction of unbound drug. The free fraction is responsible for the pharmacological action of the drug. Total (free plus bound) levels are open to misinterpretation because an apparently 'normal' level in a hypoalbuminaemic patient may hide a toxic level of free phenytoin. A conceptual corrected level can be determined, which reflects what the total phenytoin level would be if the patient had normal protein levels. To adjust for a low albumin: Adjusted phenytoin level = reported level ÷ [(0.02 × serum albumin) + 0.1] However, this equation depends on the accurate measurement of serum albumin. Some albumin assays are not reliable below 15 g/L

Action	**Patient showing toxic signs and raised level or level within range:**
	• Seek expert advice on dose reduction
	
	Patient fitting and levels low:
	• Seek advice on repeating a loading dose; and
	• Increase maintenance dose as follows:
	  – <28 μmol/L level, increase daily dose by 100 mg daily
	  – 28–48 μmol/L level, increase daily dose by 50 mg daily
	  – 48–64 μmol/L level, increase daily dose by 25 mg daily

Table 10.3 **Continued**	
Loading dose	15 mg/kg IV: maximum rate of 50 mg/minute
	Patient fitting and levels are in the therapeutic range: • Seek expert advice: patient might well need additional/ alternative therapy Before you make a dose change, seek expert advice!
NG administration and IV to oral/ng conversion	Theoretically one should take account of the different salts of the IV and oral preparation but in practice you can use a 1 to 1 conversion, but give the oral/ng as a single daily dose. Note that enteral feed reduces the absorption of phenytoin liquid so stop feed for 1 hour before and 2 hours after phenytoin administration

---

Box 10.2 Drugs that affect phenytoin levels in the body

Can *increase* levels	Can *reduce* levels
Amiodarone	Alcohol
Chloramphenicol	Antacids
Cimetidine	Carbamazepine
Clarithromycin	Rifampicin
Fluconazole	St John's Wort
Fluoxetine	Theophylline
Fluvoxamine	
Isoniazid	
Metronidazole	
Trimethoprim	
Voriconazole	

Theophylline/aminophylline

See Table 10.4 for the dosing regimen. Serum levels predict the type of adverse effects well, but are less good at predicting severity. Adverse effects of these drugs are outlined in Table 10.5.

Vancomycin

There are two methods of vancomycin therapy in use, 'conventional' and 'continuous' (Table 10.6). When samples are sent off for measurement, it is essential that they are marked with the method of use, as the interpretation of these levels is linked to this method.

Commonly prescribed drugs needing TDM

See Table 10.7.

Table 10.4 Dosing regimen for theophylline/aminophylline

Loading dose	Aminophylline 5 mg/kg IV over 20 minutes
Maintenance dose	Aminophylline 500 µg/kg/hour IV titrated to plasma levels Oral therapy depends on the brand In the obese patient, use IBW to calculate the dose, as aminophylline distributes poorly in adipose tissue
Indication	Ensure achieving therapeutic target Avoid toxicity *For IV/PO therapy:* TDM is essential, as the drug has a narrow therapeutic range
How it is done	*IV infusion:* take levels at 1 and 6 hours, repeating daily *Oral therapy:* take trough levels after 2–3 days of treatment
Interpretation	Recommended therapeutic range 55–110 µmol/L *or* 10–20 mg/L
Action	In most patients, theophylline has linear kinetics, so doubling the dose will double the serum concentration, but this is not always the case *Acute patient, with low/high level:* • Adjust dose by desired fraction *Acute patient in range:* • Repeat levels daily *Chronic patient, with low/high level:* • Having excluded a reversible cause, adjust the dose *Chronic patient in range:* • Suspected toxicity: consider a second drug or pathology causing toxic signs. You might need to stop theophylline regardless *Symptomatic patient:* • Consider alternative therapy
Important	Beware those in whom the theophylline half-life is increased, i.e. where a normal dose may cause toxicity: cardiac failure, liver failure, the elderly, those taking enzyme inhibitors (e.g. cimetidine, ciprofloxacin) Beware of those in whom the theophylline half-life is decreased, i.e. where a normal dose may be ineffective: smokers, chronic alcoholics, those taking enzyme inducers (e.g. rifampicin, phenytoin). The effect of smoking can be maintained up to 6 months after cessation Concurrent systemic salbutamol use may reduce theophylline levels
IV to oral/ng conversion	Converting aminophylline IV to aminophylline oral/ng: • Calculate 24 hours IV aminophylline requirement to attain desired level • Use a 1 to 1 conversion to convert IV to oral/ng aminophylline. For ng administration, divide the total dose into 6-hourly doses (although unlicensed, you can give the IV product down the ng tube). For oral dosing use aminophylline modified release products; divide the total dose into 12-hourly dose (round dose up or down, as the tablets are 225 mg) Converting aminophylline IV to oral/ng theophylline: • Calculate 24 hours IV aminophylline requirement to attain desired level • Multiply this by 0.79 for equivalent theophylline dose. Round up or down and convert to the nearest oral product available. Remember modified release products will block the ng tube so are not suitable

Table 10.5 Levels associated with adverse effects of aminophylline and theophylline

Level (mg/L)	Adverse reaction	Frequency (%)
<5	Usually absent	N/A
5–20	Nausea and vomiting	5–10
20–35	As above + diarrhoea, irritability, arrhythmias	25
>35	As above + seizures	80

Table 10.6 Dosing regimens for vancomycin

Conventional dosing	Usually start at 1 g IV BD For the elderly or those with low body weight: 500 mg IV BD In moderate/severe renal failure or haemofiltration: 1 g IV once and repeat dose when trough is <15 mg/L every 48–72 hours
Indication for TDM	Renally toxic and ototoxic at raised levels
How it is done	Take trough level in the morning before third or fourth dose, i.e. day 2 of treatment. Repeat levels daily.
Interpretation	*Trough level:* should be 10–15 mg/L and 15–20 for less sensitive strains of MRSA *Peak level:* these are not required

Action	*Raised trough level:*
	• 16–20 mg/L: reduce dose by 25% (e.g. to 750 mg IV BD)
	• >20 mg/L: omit drug and repeat level daily
	  – when level <15 mg/L, give 1 g IV
	  – repeat for each dose

Continuous dosing	Some units are using continuous vancomycin infusions. The main advantage is the ease of interpretation of assays
Loading dose	<70 kg: 1 g IV over 1 hour ≥70 kg: 1.25 g IV over 1 hour

Continuous IV infusion follows straight after the loading dose

	Serum creatinine (μmol/L)	Starting daily vancomycin dose	Starting infusion rate (mg/hour)
Normal renal function	<120	1500 mg	63
Impaired renal function	>120	1000 mg	42
Haemofiltration		1000 mg	42
Frequency of levels	Daily		

Table 10.6 Continued

Vancomycin level:	Dosage change required	Infusion rate adjustment
<15 mg/L	Increase the dose by 500 mg	Increase infusion rate to next level
15–25 mg/L	No change	
>25 mg/L	Decrease the dose by 500 mg*	Reduce infusion rate to next level down
>30 mg/L	Stop infusion for at least 6 hours	Restart at reduced dose agreed on ward round

*If the patient is only receiving 500 mg/day, the dose should be decreased to 250 mg/day.
Acknowledgement to Guy's and St Thomas's Critical Care Unit

Table 10.7 Commonly prescribed drugs requiring therapeutic drugs monitoring

Drug	Half-life (hours)	Target range	When to sample	Sampling notes
Carbamazepine	Chronic therapy: 5–27	17–51 µmol/L 4–12 mg/L	Trough level after 2–4 weeks	Aim for higher end-of-range if monotherapy Half-life decreases with chronic therapy
Ciclosporin	Neoral preps: 8.4 (5–18) Sandimum preps: 19 (10–27)	Very broad depending on indication, typically 200–600 µg/L (168–498 nanomol/L). Should not exceed toxic levels of 600 µg/L (498 nanomol/L)	Trough	Check with primary team for the required target range. Beware of many drug interactions. Note there are two brands of ciclosporin (Neoral PO and Sandimmun PO and IV). Care is required with conversion
Lithium	18	0.4–1.3 mmol/L 15–48 mg/L	12 hours postdose	Desired level varies with indication
Phenobarbital	120	65–172 µmol/L 15–40 mg/L	Anytime after 3–4 weeks, due to long half-life	Poor correlation between level and response
Sodium valproate	8–15	350–700 µmol/L 50–100 mg/L	Take trough level after 2–4 days	Correlation between level and efficacy less reliable